# ZERO SUGAR DETOX

DISCOVER HOW YOU CAN OVERCOME YOUR
SILENT ADDICTION, CRUSH YOUR CRAVINGS, AND
BURN FAT EFFORTLESSLY IN THE PROCESS

CODY SMITH

# CONTENTS

*Read First*     7

*Introduction*     9

1. Why Sugar Is Destroying Your Health     15
2. A Drug for the Whole Family     32
3. The Sweet Life Without Sugar     40
4. Why A Detox is Your Best Option     50
5. What to Expect During Your Detox     57
6. Foods That Will Ruin Your Detox the Moment You Eat Them     71
7. What to Eat to Crush Your Detox From Day 1     92
8. The Most Crucial Step: Accountability     108
9. When Craving Rears Its Ugly Face     120
10. Putting It All Together     130

*Bonus Chapter: The Wiggle Factor*     145

*Afterword*     149

*Join the Facebook Group!*     151

*Who is Cody Smith?*     153

*References*     155

information contained within this document, including, but not limited to, errors, omissions, or inaccuracies.

Thank you for choosing this book to guide you on kicking sugar to the curb through a powerful detox. As an appreciation, I would love to give you the Zero Sugar Detox Starter Kit
as a FREE gift.
The Zero Sugar Detox Starter Kit includes:
**The Zero Sugar Detox Summary:** We don't always have time to read an entire book so I've created a quick summary of each chapter with all of the juiciest info.
**5 stupid easy sugar-free recipes that are delicious, dummy proof, and will send your taste buds to the moon! Recipes with sugar won't stand a chance after you've tried just one of these.**
You are also going to get a FREE PDF copy of my

latest and high anticipated book, The Wiggle Factor. What you'll discover in that book will literally allow you to kiss dieting goodbye and still drop that extra weight (even if nothing else has worked).

Go to this URL:

https://fearpunchingcody.com/zerosugardetoxkit

or use the QR code for your free gifts.

You can also simply text **DETOXSUGAR** to (678) 506-7543 to download your free starter kit along with a free copy of my latest book.

A high sugar diet is not healthy for anyone, and this includes you. But what most people don't know is that this seemingly sweet substance increases the risk of heart disease, obesity, and diabetes, along with other chronic diseases. In fact, according to an estimate which was initially presented in a scientific meeting in 2013, it was proposed that sugary beverages alone are the cause of 184,000 deaths around the globe each year!

These deaths are caused by cancer, heart disease, and diabetes, all of which scientists say can be attributed directly to the consumption of sweetened beverages. This is a high fatality rate, and nobody wants to become part of a statistic like that. To compound the problem, sugar is everywhere and very easy to get addicted to, since we are naturally attuned to love it. The downsides of sugar are proof enough that excessive consumption is simply not worth the risk.

Many people make a vow to themselves to limit the amount of sugar they consume. Some of them have been able to successfully accomplish this, while others always find themselves right back where they began—back to the sugar monster! If you belong to the latter group, and you have tried everything you could but just can't seem to get it right, then you are in luck! By purchasing this book, you have put yourself ahead of many others in the quest for a solution to this problem. The difference between those who were able to get it right and those who went right back is that they were armed with the correct information, which you will also be presented within this book.

What you need is to break away from sugar completely by doing a detox to help you entirely flush it out of your system, along with that pesky addiction that comes with it. You need to break the dependence your body has developed that makes it yearn for sugar. You need to reset your brain back to the state where it did not crave as much sugar as you have conditioned it to.

A true sugar detox does not mean you simply stop eating sugar. This is where many people tend to get it wrong. In addition to knowing which foods to avoid, you need to also acquire the right mindset and to learn how to be accountable in order for this journey to be a successful one.

Breaking away from sugar addiction is not exactly a walk in the park, considering most of the meals we consume today consist of profound amounts of added sugar, even going beyond the most obvious ones. Sugar has become so abundant in our food system that it's difficult to avoid it. What makes it worse is that, many people run back into the inviting arms of sugar when the cravings come or when they are dealing with a few withdrawal symptoms. This is a major reason why many people who have tried quitting sugar without the right guidance tend to find themselves back where they started. I'll help you avoid the cravings and withdrawal symptoms stemming from a lifetime of excessive sugar consumption.

Giving up this pleasurable substance comes with numerous benefits in your life. In return for your efforts, you regain control of your weight and get more rejuvenating sleep than what you are used to.

But that's not the ultimate benefit, as getting rid of sugar also reduces your risk of many severe health problems such as heart disease, kidney disease, and even diabetes and dementia. Lastly, you will fully leverage the benefit of enjoying a life filled with happiness, since excess sugar is tied to mental health issues, including depression and anxiety.

All of this and much more is what you will discover in this book. I have laid everything out in an easy to understand manner, and I am confident that if you follow the plan that is mapped out in this book

you will transform your life in a fantastic way. Over the years, I have helped many people to completely eliminate sugar from their lives, and once they started experiencing the benefits of a life without excess sugar, none of them wanted to ever go back. In fact, many of them continue to reach out to me to show their appreciation. You too can be one of them. You can kick sugar to the curb and experience the life you have been missing out on.

As you know, time waits for no one. This is a decision you need to make today. The more sugar you consume, the more danger you put yourself in. You will continue to crave for more, and soon you will need to increase the amount of sugar you consume to get the same kind of "high" you are used to. This is how many people get addicted, and breaking away becomes an uphill battle.

Even with the right support guide, any restrictive diet or detox can be difficult to implement, which is why I've included a bonus chapter in the back of the book to show you how to make this work for you. If at any point you are reading the book and start to think *I don't know if I can do this*—and chances are you will—turn to the bonus chapter. I'll show you how to instantly make any restrictive diet, including this detox, less punishing, more practical, and flexible enough to fit your unique lifestyle while still seeing results. This is my promise to you to ensure you have everything you need to be successful, even with something as hard as breaking away from sugar.

If you are serious about banishing sugar from your life, you need to start now. You deserve to enjoy a healthy lifestyle. Do it for yourself, and for those who care about you. You deserve happiness, so you should go all out to get it.

Let's dive right in!

# WHY SUGAR IS DESTROYING YOUR HEALTH

I s sugar inherently bad for you?

The simple answer is both yes and no.

No, because sugar does offer your body some legitimate benefits; and yes, because if you consume an excessive amount, it's detrimental to your health. This is because when there is adequate energy in our bodies, it stores any surplus sugar for future use by converting it into fat. However, in the age we live in now, most of us are eating more sugar than the energy we burn. This means the major problem lies in the quantity and type of sugar we consume. Let's take a closer look at this.

**Types of Sugar**

**Sugar** can be broken down into two main categories:

- **Natural Sugars**: This includes the kind of sugar you find in dairy products like cheese and milk, known as lactose. It also includes those you find in starchy vegetables and fruits. These foods consist of vital nutrients that can help prevent ailments and keep your body healthy. Natural sources of sugar take more time to digest and help you feel full for longer periods. In general, they don't cause a spike in the blood-sugar level of your body.

- **Refined/Processed Sugars:** This is the most common kind of sugar you see in grocery stores today. It is extracted from natural sources through a process that rids it of all its nutrients and fibers, leaving an unnaturally high form of concentrated sugar molecules. This high concentration is broken down and digested by the body faster, and causes an unnatural spike in blood sugar and insulin levels. You'll discover soon why controlling these two factors, blood sugar and insulin, is the key to reversing disease, low energy, and weight gain.

While our ancestors only consumed sugar sparingly when they were able to find natural sources during certain seasons, our diet nowadays is filled with refined and processed sugar on a daily basis. Most snacks, cereals, and beverages come with tons of added sugar, which leads to people consuming more than their body can healthily metabolize.

**Sugar Is Not All Bad**

In reality, sugar is not all bad. In fact, it's crucial to the survival of humans, as sugar in the form of glucose is a vital source of energy for your muscles, nervous system and brain. Glucose fuels all of the cells of your body, but it needs the help of insulin to keep your blood-sugar level stable. When your blood sugar rises, which typically happens after you eat, your body releases insulin to handle the excess amount. It does this by acting like a key for a lock to open up cells allowing them to accept glucose and use as fuel.

However, our bodies only need so much of this fuel at any given moment. Once our cells have all they need, the insulin then tells the liver to convert the excess glucose into glycogen, which is simply a form of glucose that can be stored by the body. Glycogen is mainly stored in the liver and muscles and is easily converted later to glucose for quick energy. Because of this, our bodies will always prioritize burning glycogen as fuel over fat storage, which is not as easily accessible.

Regardless of the benefits it provides, you need to be cautious about how much sugar you consume. All of the benefits we have discussed come only when you consume natural sugar, and in moderation. If you fail to do so, it can lead to damaging effects.

**The Problem**

There is no doubt that many individuals consume excess sugar, especially processed sugar. In America alone, individuals consume around 57 pounds of added sugar every year. This is equivalent to an average of 71 grams (or 17 teaspoons) of added sugar every day. This is almost three times more than the recommended ceiling of 25 grams (six teaspoons) daily for women, and 38 grams (nine teaspoons) for men, as outlined by the American Heart Association. All of this excess sugar is delivering a serious blow to our health and waistlines.

Now let's look into what happens to your body when you consume too much added sugar.

## THE NEGATIVE EFFECTS OF EATING TOO MUCH SUGAR

At this point, you now understand that sugar is indeed beneficial to your body since glucose is essential for our survival; but when it's not consumed in moderation, it proves to be problematic. In this modern age, eating sugar in excess is very difficult to avoid, considering the bountiful amount infused in processed meals, soft drinks, and other modern foods. Even meals that claim to be sugar-free have some level of added sugar to give them the taste that people have come to expect. It's simply too much for our bodies to handle in a healthy way.

So, how does the body handle it? Below, we will be taking a comprehensive look at some of the negative impacts of a high sugar diet on your health.

**Weight Gain**

Your body can store about a day's worth of glycogen, to later be used as quick fuel. Once your body has enough glycogen for the short term, insulin tells your liver to instead convert glucose into fat, which is used for long term storage in case the body runs out of glycogen.

What's interesting about this process is that not only does insulin tell the body to store excess sugar as fat, insulin also tells the body not to burn that fat if there's glycogen to burn instead. This is a source of a lot of confusion for people when they try to lose weight.

With our Western diet which is high in carbs, typically in the form of added sugars, we are constantly replenishing our glycogen reserves, which means we never touch our fat reserves. Even if you go to the gym and burn 500 calories, in reality, you burned 500 calories worth of glycogen, not fat. If during or after the workout you consumed any source of carbohydrates like a sports drink, yogurt, oatmeal, protein bar, etc., all you did was replenish your glycogen levels and accomplished nothing.

How frustrating is that!?

This is why it is so important to get your blood sugar and insulin levels under control, so you can actually tap into your fat storage as fuel, which will lead to real and permanent weight loss. If you stay on the track of eating a high-carb, high-sugar diet, your body has no choice but to keep storing it as fat, and never getting a chance to burn it. This is the fast track to obesity and even worse health problems.

If this wasn't bad enough, in the past 50 years a new type of sweetener has entered our food system in mass, which is even sweeter and cheaper than processed sugar. This is none other than the notorious high fructose corn syrup (HFCS). Because it's sweeter and so darn cheap, food manufacturers put it in practically everything you can imagine—from soda to bread, soup, and even pasta sauce.

What's interesting about fructose is how it's processed in the body compared to glucose. Glucose is a source of fuel for every cell in the body, but fructose is processed almost solely by the liver, and is therefore almost immediately converted into fat. And not just any type of fat, but what's called visceral fat, which is fat that hugs the organs around your midsection.

Ever heard of a beer belly? This is the name given to people who drink excessive levels of alcohol, which produces proportionally more fat storage around their midsection compared to the rest of their body. The reason for this is the way the body processes the ethanol in alcoholic beverages, which is a carbohy-drate. The liver is mainly in charge of handling excess ethanol, and does so by converting it into visceral fat. Is this starting to sound familiar?

If you've guessed that there is a correlation between how your body processes ethanol and fructose, you are absolutely correct. The process is almost identi-cal. Instead of having a beer belly, consumers of high levels of fructose end up with what's called a sugar belly.

You might be thinking, *but wait, isn't fructose found in fruit?*

Yes, it's found naturally in fruit, but in reasonable quantities and surrounded by fiber, which slows down the digestion of sugar in the body and helps with converting it more efficiently. But with our highly processed diets, we unknowingly consume high levels of fructose in the form of HFCS, day in and day out. We bombard our livers with so much fructose that it has no choice but to store it as visceral fat.

Putting it all together, our diet is constantly restoring our glycogen level, storing excess glucose as fat, converting fructose into visceral fat, and preventing us from ever using fat as fuel. That's a recipe for disaster.

**Tooth Decay**

Sugar can interact with bacteria in the teeth. When this happens, it creates acids that damage and degrade the tooth enamel, which eventually causes your teeth to rot.

Contrary to the common belief that sugar causes a cavity, it's actually the acid created when sugar reacts with the bacteria on your tooth surface. Normally our teeth are fully equipped to handle this occasional chemical reaction; however, our constant modern consumption of sugar at every meal, along with snacks throughout the day, never gives our teeth a break.

**Type 2 Diabetes**

Excess sugar consumption leads to weight gain, which is a major contributing factor to type 2 diabetes. In fact, it's categorized as one of the leading causes of the condition.

When you consistently consume sugar in high amounts, it often leads to insulin resistance. If you remember from before, insulin is responsible for the regulation of your blood-sugar level when it gets too high. Chronically high blood sugar and resulting chronically high insulin levels create a condition where your body doesn't respond to insulin as it should. In essence, your cells are less sensitive to insulin, and now need more of it to do the same job as before. As a result, people develop type 2 diabetes and require insulin shots to keep their blood sugar under control.

Unfortunately, adding more insulin to your system "fixes" merely one issue; counteracting the high blood sugar, instead of addressing the underlying problem of a diet high in sugar. Insulin does help lower your blood sugar, but that sugar doesn't just magically disappear. It gets stored as fat, because that's what insulin does. And what is a major contributing factor to developing type 2 diabetes? Weight gain. This creates a disgusting cycle that unfortunately gets worse and worse until you finally deal with the source of the problem; what you eat.

**Heart Disease**

Since the 1970s, saturated fat has been identified as the main cause of concern for developing heart disease. Researchers observed that peoples' arteries were being clogged with a buildup of low-density lipoprotein (LDL) cholesterol, the so-called "bad" cholesterol. It was believed that the source of all this "bad" cholesterol was saturated fat. This was partially true but gave rise to some very misleading and wrong assumptions.

It's true that consuming saturated fats raises LDL cholesterol in your bloodstream, but assuming this is the root cause of heart disease is questionable and far too simplistic. This is where the initial research got it all wrong.

LDL cholesterol, like high-density lipoprotein (HDL) cholesterol, plays a very important role in your body. What many people don't know is that there are actually seven different types of LDL cholesterol. Types one and two share a similar makeup (known as "Pattern A LDL") which is non-oxidized and completely harmless. Types 3 through 7 are Pattern B LDL, which is oxidized. It's these Pattern B LDLs that end up clogging arteries.

Guess which type shows up when you eat saturated fat?

Pattern A. The harmless LDL.

Guess what shows up when you eat lots of carbohydrates (aka sugar)?

Pattern B. The harmful LDL.

The liver can process Pattern A LDL all day long. It has a special protein that acts as an all-access ID card to get into the liver. But if this ID card gets damaged, the liver can't recognize the LDL any longer and treats it as a foreign substance. How does this protein get damaged? The answer is simple: glucose.

Glucose can actually bind to this protein, damage it, and turn it into oxidized Pattern B LDL. This oxidized LDL, which can no longer be pulled out of the bloodstream through the liver, must now be dealt with through other means. Unfortunately, this "other means" is what ultimately leads to heart disease.

The body doesn't want Pattern B LDL just circulating in the bloodstream forever, so it uses cells called macrophages that gobble them up inside the wall of the blood vessel. Eventually, the buildup of these macrophages will start to clog the blood vessels, resulting in heart disease as we know it.

Saturated fat was never the problem, and neither was LDL cholesterol. The true culprit was sugar.

**Liver Disease**

Remember our discussion on fructose and how the liver turns it into visceral fat that hugs our organs? Some of that fat is deposited inside the liver itself. In the past, a fatty liver was typically associated with excessive alcohol consumption, which would cause fatty liver disease. But you can develop the exact same thing thanks to good ole' fructose.

The more weight we gain, the harder it gets for us to fulfill our daily functions. The same goes for the liver. I don't know about you, but I prefer a liver in full working order.

## Alzheimer's and Dementia (a.k.a. "Type 3 Diabetes")

Who knew there could be such a thing? If type 2 diabetes is caused by your cells becoming insulin resistant, the currently proposed "type 3 diabetes" is where your brain becomes insulin resistant.

Your brain is a glucose goblin. It loves the sweet stuff and needs a ton of it as fuel to fully operate. But what happens when the brain becomes resistant to insulin, which is the key to allowing glucose to enter brain cells? Now the brain isn't getting all the fuel it needs to fully operate. The theory is that as the brain becomes more and more insulin resistant, the lack of fuel over time is what leads to conditions such as dementia and possibly even Alzheimer's.

Has this been fully proven to be the case? No. Is current research pointing towards this being the case? It looks that way, but more research needs to be done.

For those who are completely opposed to the idea that a type 3 diabetes exists, and that overconsumption of sugar is a probable cause for conditions such as dementia or Alzheimer's, I have a question for you. If insulin resistance can cause devastating harm to the body, why would the brain, as glucose hungry and dependent as it is, be immune to the same level of harm?

A common current theory is that the brain is the last level of defense against a life of high sugar consumption. When you look at children who lacked adequate food during their development years, their heads are disproportionately larger than the rest of their body. This is caused by the body doing everything it can to conserve the brain, especially during years of starvation, while foregoing the rest of the body. I believe a similar conservation of the brain happens when eating a diet high in sugar year in and year out. The body will experience the consequences of insulin resistance years before the brain ever will. This is why I think symptoms of dementia or Alzheimer's typically don't show up until our golden years. The body has done everything it could to protect the brain until it can no longer, and all is lost.

KEY POINTS

In this chapter, you have discovered the major types of sugars: natural sugars from fruits and dairy; and refined sugar, which is the highly processed type.

- Broken down into its main parts, refined sugar is made up of fructose and glucose, and we consume an insane amount of it every year thanks to the modern Western diet.
- Fructose is cheaper and sweeter than glucose, which is why you can find it in almost all processed foods, usually in the form of high fructose corn syrup. Fructose, even though it's found naturally in fruit, is processed very similarly to how ethanol from alcohol is processed; by the liver. The liver, for the most part, turns fructose

straight into visceral fat, the type that hugs the organs around our midsection. This can lead to a similar appearance of an alcoholic's beer belly except, in this case, it's a sugar belly.

- Glucose, on the other hand, is used to fuel every cell in the body, but it cannot do that without insulin. Insulin is used by the body to open cells, so they can receive glucose as fuel. Excess glucose is converted to glycogen, which is the storage form of glucose kept in the liver and muscles. Your body reserves about a day's worth of calories as glycogen. Excess glucose beyond that is converted into fat.

- If you have glycogen reserves available, your body will not use your fat as fuel. This is why dieting is so freakin' hard. You could be busting your butt in the gym, eating what you're "supposed" to eat, and still not lose weight. If your diet is high in carbs, even healthy carbs like fruit or whole grains, your body will keep restoring its glycogen levels and never tap into its fat storage. Sugar is what turns healthy "Pattern A" LDL cholesterol into oxidized "Pattern B" LDL cholesterol, which is what clogs arteries and leads to heart disease.

- Excess sugar intake leads to the cells of your body becoming insulin resistant, meaning your body now needs more insulin to do the same job it did before. It is this that leads to type 2 diabetes, and possibly dementia and Alzheimer's, which a growing number of researchers now classify as "type 3 diabetes".

Regardless of the source, sugar in high doses can absolutely wreck your body, whether it comes from apple pie or just plain apples. So why do we find it so difficult to give up? We'll explore the troubling answer to that question in the next chapter.

## A DRUG FOR THE WHOLE FAMILY

We all know sugar is bad for us, but there's something about labeling it as a drug that just seems far-fetched to many. When you look at a picture of someone battling a meth addiction and compare that to a child enjoying a piece of candy, the comparison tends to destroy any validity of sugar being as harmful as a drug. Nor have I ever given money to a homeless person and worried that they might spend it on cake. But there are some very unique characteristics of sugar that help it fit under the category of a drug and that's its effect on the reward center of the brain.

**We Are Born to Love Sugar, and Corporations Know It**

Humans are genetically hardwired to prefer sweet flavors. We consume even just a little bit of it, and it lights up our brain's pleasure sensors, prompting us to do that again. This genetic disposition helped our ancestors survive because sweet foods such as fruits served as a great source of quick energy. It was more challenging back then to find concentrated sugar sources, so it was beneficial to crave sugar in the little amounts they could access them.

But with the improvement in agricultural technology, not only has fruit become abundantly available all year long, but so have highly concentrated processed sugars and sweeteners. What was once a scarce resource is now available inexpensively to everyone any time of the day.

Now you can find sugar in almost any type of food. It is of course present in the more obvious foods like soda, cake, and candy; but you can also find it in condiments, bread, crackers, and other places where you would least expect it. In fact, according to a report from UCSF's SugarScience.org, 76 percent of packaged and processed foods contain added sugar. Why? Because food manufacturers know we love it. It's a cheap way to make food light up your brain's pleasure sensors so that you, the consumer, will come back for more. Tons of research and development dollars are spent every year to pinpoint the exact amount of sugar to add to a product to ensure it flies off the shelf. These corporations are trying to engineer their products to determine what's called the "bliss point," the industry term to describe the minimum level of sweetness needed to make a customer addicted.

What used to help us survive is now being used against us, to trick us into consuming an excess amount of sugar beyond what our bodies can deal with in a healthy manner.

**Sugar Is Addictive Like a Drug**

Research has shown that sugar causes the same kind of stimulation in the brain as addictive drugs do. Therefore, the sudden cutoff of sugar results in the same kind of withdrawal and dependence. If meth stimulates the reward center of the brain like fireworks going off, then sugar is more like a bonfire, in that it's not as flashy or intense but you can keep it burning all day long, every day of the year. And you can easily add gasoline to the fire with a soda, a bowl of cereal, or "healthy" yogurt.

With time, your tolerance for sugar increases, and

you will need to go past your normal threshold to keep the flame burning as high as before. This happens because any time you consume excess sugar, there is a huge amount of dopamine released. Over time, your dopamine receptors start to become less and less responsive. As a result, you're forced to consume even more sugar to feel the same way.

**Sugar Makes You Hungrier Faster**

As if addiction wasn't enough to make it difficult to quit sugar, it gets worse.

Have you ever been in the middle of eating a high carb meal and thought, *How am I not full yet? How on earth can I keep eating? What is wrong with me?* You can feel your stomach reaching maximum capacity to the point of discomfort, and yet you feel you could just keep going.

I'm happy to tell you there's nothing wrong with you. What's wrong is your diet, which is literally hindering your body from turning off your appetite.

That's because sugar messes with your leptin hormone levels. This is the "I've had enough food" hormone that tells you when you are satisfied. It is made by fat cells as a response to the deposition of energy. Basically, your fat is literally trying to help you not be fat. Leptin is pushed into the bloodstream and finds its way to the numerous organs in your body to inform them that the amount of energy available is adequate. In essence, leptin controls your appetite. If your brain fails to see a signal from the leptin, then it assumes that you are still hungry and need to take in more food.

Insulin blocks leptin signals to the brain; and so if you experience an overload of insulin, it means your brain never gets the signal that you've had enough. This happens naturally two times in your life: when you're going through puberty and when you're pregnant. It appears the body would like for you to keep putting on weight during times of intense growth, or when you're supporting growth for reproduction, even if you've eaten enough to normally feel "full."

But artificially, you're able to create the same biological response with a diet high in sugar. The result of this is that you continue to eat and eat, never feeling satisfied, since your leptin receptors have basically been turned off. When the sugar wears off and you crash, you turn back to sugar as a means to feel better, resulting in a never-ending cycle of literally feeding your addiction.

And speaking of crashes...

**The Dreaded Sugar Crash**

When we consume unnaturally high amounts of sugar, we unnaturally spike our blood sugar, experience an unnaturally high dopamine response, feel unnaturally amazing, and end with an unnatural drop in blood sugar, known to most of us as the crash, and typically described as feeling lethargic, fatigued, and irritable.

A dramatic crash in blood sugar also causes your body to release adrenaline (the fight-or-flight hormone) and cortisol (the stress hormone) to try and stabilize your blood-sugar level. So not only do you feel a lack of energy during the crash, but you also feel stressed and anxious. It's during this time that you'll start looking for a pick-me-up to feel "normal" again.

Sound familiar?

And people wonder why they feel like emotional eaters. Our diet is causing an emotional, stress, and anxiety-infused roller coaster that we experience multiple times per day, every day of the year because we continuously turn to sugar-loaded food to fix a problem it caused to begin with.

## KEY POINTS

In this chapter you discovered why sugar is so addictive and so hard to give up.

- **We are born to love it:** Because our ancestors got quick energy from sugar, it is embedded deep within us to love it. As soon as you taste it, the brain registers it as a pleasurable substance that we can't seem to get enough of.
- **It is very addictive**: Sugar urges your brain to release dopamine, which is a feel-good chemical, similar to what many feel during drug use. When you no longer consume it, you can experience withdrawal symptoms similar to drug withdrawal, because your brain has become dependent on it. Not to mention, you can grow a tolerance to sugar, which means you need more and more to get the same dopamine release as you did before.
- **You can find it almost everywhere**: Processed sugar is in almost everything we consume these days—from the most obvious culprits like soda and candy, down to

surprising ones like whole grain bread, rice, oatmeal, and salad dressings.

- **It causes a ravenous appetite**: Insulin, the hormone to deal with all that sugar intake, actively turns off your leptin signals so that you keep eating and never feel satisfied.
- **It causes a nasty sugar crash**: The high highs inevitably lead to low lows in your blood-sugar levels. These drastic swings cause you to feel low in energy, stressed and anxious, causing you to turn back to sugar to feel "better" again.

When you have had enough and finally do quit sugar, you will have to deal with withdrawals in order to completely free yourself. There is no easy way out of quitting sugar, as you will need to put in the effort involved. We will be taking a more detailed look at this in chapter 5; but for now, let's next examine all the great things that come from a life without sugar.

## THE SWEET LIFE WITHOUT SUGAR

Y ou've already discovered a lot about what sugar does to the body and ultimately your health. You've discovered how high insulin levels, the result of consuming lots of sugar, are literally stopping you from using your stored fat as fuel. You've uncovered the very addictive nature of sugar, how it's stopping your brain from registering the leptin signal to control your appetite, and how the inevitable sugar crash leaves you feeling emotional, stressed, and anxious before turning back to sugar to "fix" the problem.

Luckily, getting away from sugar can allow you to access your stored fat, regulate a healthy appetite, end your addiction, and relieve you of the endless highs and lows that come with it. In this chapter, you're going to discover a few more shocking benefits of getting sugar out of your life. Then you'll be ready to dive into the details and get your sugar detox off to a great start.

## Better Skin

They say that the skin is an outward reflection of your internal health (or lack thereof). Sugar intake can literally wreck you from the inside out, but luckily you have a lot to gain from letting go of the sweet stuff. From minimizing acne to slowing down the aging process and reducing wrinkles, your skin will enjoy the amazing benefits of giving up sugar. Let's cover some of these benefits in more detail.

### Slowing Down the Aging Process

Remember when we discussed how sugar oxidizes LDL cholesterol and ultimately causes heart disease? Sugar has a very similar effect on other cells in the body too, like skin cells. Sugar responds to the body's proteins and changes their structure to create advanced glycation end products (AGEs), which speed up the process of aging.

Sugar isn't so sweet when it's trying to steal your looks. AGEs cause wrinkles, eye bags, and dull, saggy skin. The more sugar you consume, the more AGEs are created in your body, making you look way older than your actual age.

However, when you give up sugar, it makes elastin and collagen more resilient, radiant, supple, and elastic. By giving up sugar, fewer AGEs are created, which in turn slows down the aging process.

**Reducing Acne and Psoriasis**

When your body processes sugar, it quickly raises your insulin levels, thereby triggering inflammation. Inflammation then results in whiteheads, black-heads, and other forms of acne, all of which affect the way you look and even your self-confidence. Getting rid of sugar from your diet can help you deal with acne .

However, acne is not the only result of inflammation; it's also been observed to be one of the major triggers of psoriasis. This is a skin condition that hastens the life cycle of the skin cells, causing a rapid buildup of new cells on the skin surface, and an increased supply of blood. The additional skin cells cause itching and sometimes excruciating red patches and scales, while the increase in blood results in redness and swelling.

When you give up sugar, the acne and psoriasis

flare-ups you experience won't be as frequent or critical.

## Making Your Skin More Resistant to the Sun

As you know, the consumption of sugar results in the production of AGEs. AGEs are harmful to the antioxidant enzymes in the body, and these enzymes keep your skin safe from the dangerous UV rays in sunlight. This means sugar can cause the skin to be less resistant to the sun's damaging effects.

To put it simply, getting rid of sugar in your diet makes your skin less prone to damage from UV rays.

## Better Sleep

Studies have proven that taking in excess sugar is associated with disrupted and uncomfortable sleep. This was further supported by a study that was carried out in 2016, consisting of healthy volunteers put in one of two groups. The first group was allowed to consume any type and portion size of a meal they desired, leading to diets with a tremendous amount of fat and sugar, while the other group was on a diet that focused on fiber and excluded sugar and fats. The researchers observed that those who consumed meals filled with sugar slept deeply for less time. They also took more time to fall asleep and woke up more frequently throughout the night. Sleeping is crucial for the healing and physical restoration of the body, as well as maintaining a functional immune system and a healthy metabolism.

Uncomfortable and poor sleep also has an impact on sugar consumption. When you are exhausted from not getting enough sleep, you have a higher tendency to consume more junk food for a quick energy boost.

If during the day you consume high levels of sugar during a meal or snack, your blood sugar spikes and eventually crashes. Do you remember what your body does to try and stabilize your sugar levels?

It releases a dose of adrenaline.

Now imagine your evening dinner or a late-night snack is a high-carb, sugar-spiking explosion so common in the typical American diet. Your blood sugar will spike, fueling you with quick energy, which makes it harder to go to sleep. Eventually, the sugar surge will end, and you'll be able to drift off to sleep, but not for long. Soon after the crash, your body will release adrenaline (the fight-or-flight hormone) while you're sleeping.

Imagine the amount of restful sleep you're getting with adrenaline coursing through your body. Your body's attempt to stabilize your blood sugar will either wake you up or, at the very least, pull you out of deep sleep. This deep sleep is what makes you feel rested when you wake up in the morning. Without enough time in deep sleep, you'll wake up feeling like a hot pile of garbage, as if you didn't sleep at all. Often the quickest "solution" to this problem is to grab something loaded with sugar in the morning, to get a quick boost in energy to start the day.

And the cycle starts all over again.

If you're waking up exhausted every morning because of your sugar consumption, something is terribly wrong. That may be your normal, but that is *not* normal.

**Stable Energy Levels**

As you can imagine, getting truly restful sleep plays a huge role in your energy throughout the day. We've all experienced a terrible night's sleep that resulted in feeling groggy as if you're spending half the next day trying to fully wake up. Conversely, we've all experienced a blissful night's sleep where you wake up feeling alive and energetic.

Because your sleep quality plays a role in your energy the next day, and sugar impacts your sleep quality, then it follows that sugar has a role in determining your energy. Getting sugar out of your life will allow you to have a consistent, restful sleep, which in turn will allow you to have the consistent energy levels to handle whatever life throws at you.

Furthermore, when you take sugar out of your diet, you also take the sugar spikes and crashes out of your life as well. No more dealing with the extreme highs and lows in your energy levels. You'll surprise yourself when 2 PM comes around and you feel perfectly fine to tackle the rest of the afternoon, while everyone else is reaching for a fourth cup of coffee and sugary snacks to get them through the end of the workday.

### All-Around Happiness

Let's face it, sugar brings a momentary feeling of pleasure into your life unlike anything else. Giving up sugar feels like you'll be losing a source of happiness that cannot be replaced. What you may not realize is that you have given up a great deal in exchange for this short-term pleasure.

You've given up your ability to use your stored fat as

fuel, which has resulted in weight gain, unwanted pounds, and the poor body image that comes with it.

You've increased your chances of developing heart disease by clogging up your arteries with damaged LDL cholesterol.

You've given up control over your appetite, further feeding an addiction to sugar.

You've given up control over what you eat and instead, you're letting what you eat control you.

You've given up truly restful sleep.

You've given up stable energy throughout the day.

Giving up all of that for sugar seems crazy because it is. No one in their right mind would intentionally give all of that up, but we do it every single day with the choices we make in what we eat.

If you ask me, this isn't a balanced trade-off. You've gotten the short end of the stick. But you can take it all back.

True happiness comes from a life that's a joy to live over the long term. Happiness is not found in short, momentary spikes in pleasure that leave you worse off in the end.

Take your life back by taking sugar out of it.

## KEY POINTS

Giving up sugar offers you a range of benefits:

- **It is better for your skin:** Removing sugar from your diet helps you get rid of wrinkles and eye bags Because sugar creates toxic AGEs in the body, which hasten the aging process, you get to enjoy a youthful look for longer when you give up a diet high in sugar.
- **It helps you sleep better:** A no-sugar diet can help you get better sleep by ensuring you fall asleep much quicker and sleep more soundly. What's more, you wake up feeling completely refreshed instead of feeling like you have not had enough sleep.
- **Stable energy levels:** Taking sugar out of your diet can help you maintain stable energy levels, as opposed to them constantly spiking and crashing.
- **It leads to all-around happiness:** Giving up sugar may feel like you're giving up on a source of pleasure in your life, but it's easy to forget all the other sources of pleasure that it

has caused you to give up gradually over time—things like a healthy weight, heart, and liver, not to mention restful sleep, stable energy, and full control over appetite along with what you eat.

You have so much to gain and so little to lose by giving up sugar. This next chapter will show you exactly how to kick sugar to the curb once and for all.

# WHY A DETOX IS YOUR BEST OPTION

By now, you understand just how damaging excess sugar can be for your health. In this section, we will look into what a sugar detox is and how to start one. But before jumping right in, let's talk about what a sugar detox entails.

## What is a Sugar Detox?

Many people believe a sugar detox only involves getting rid of sugary treats in your diet. While cutting down on sweets is a significant step, other things need to be considered. Many foods have added sugar, aside from the more obvious offenders like soda or chocolate. Some foods are marketed as healthy meals, but they have significant amounts of sugar in them. Many of these meals consist of simple carbohydrates, which end up metabolizing into glucose in our bodies.

The reality is that many foods that we use as healthy weight-loss options are the culprits behind our weight gain. In order to start combating this, we need to wean our body off of its sugar dependency. A sugar detox involves ridding your body of sugar and then avoiding it entirely, even from natural sources like fruit.

This detox may sound a little extreme, but if you have consumed a high carb diet for a long time, you probably have developed a tolerance to sugar, and potentially even an addiction. Most people don't realize just how dependent they are on sugar until they remove sugar from their diet. Luckily, a sugar detox provides a structure for you to change your eating habits.

### How Long Should a Sugar Detox Last?

The length of a sugar detox is determined by how dependent you have become on it. But generally speaking, you need to give yourself at least three days for the detox, and you can extend that length depending on what fits best for you.

Before diving in, you will need to consider your

schedule. Ideally, you should try to avoid days that you will have food plans with your friends or loved ones. For the sugar detox to work, you will want to eat mostly homemade meals. This allows you to be in control of the ingredients so that you can ensure you are eating sugar-free meals.

When it involves sugar detox plans, there are three common time-frames people use:

- 3 days
- 1-2 weeks
- 1 month

The three-day plan can be a great option after periods where you have consumed a considerable amount of sugar. Good examples of this may be after a vacation, Christmas, or other holidays. In this plan, you drop sugar cold turkey to quickly reset your body and rid it of the unhealthy sugars you may have consumed.

The one to two-week plan requires you to plan and strategize. However, it is an ideal option for anyone who wants to permanently reduce their sugar levels. It also is great for those who are feeling low on energy and have added excess weight.

The one month plan is the most challenging of the options, but certainly not impossible. This option best suits those who have become excessively overweight and are unable to get their weight and cravings in check.

## Should You Do A Cold Turkey or Gradual Detox Plan?

Because of the addictive nature of sugar, I personally recommend going cold turkey. Even though doing a gradual detox where you slowly cut back on sugar is more manageable, it is less beneficial in the long run. Anyone who has tried cutting back on sugar knows it's hard to stop eating it once you have even a small bit. You may have intentions of eating just one cookie, but quickly one becomes an entire sleeve and you're just getting warmed up.

When you go cold turkey and immediately cut off sugar, your body is forced to adapt quickly to living without it. It also means your withdrawal symptoms won't linger around for as long. For this to be effective, you need to cut all forms of sugar out of your diet completely.

## Our Goal: The Two-Week Cold Turkey Plan

Like I stated earlier, the best option is dependent on

your body type and level of tolerance, so it will vary from person to person. The ideal time period for you is also dependent on what you hope to achieve during the sugar detox. Still, the above plans are the most commonly recommended for anyone who is looking to rid their body of sugar altogether. My personal suggestion is for a complete two-week sugar detox.

A two-week plan is a great balance between the shorter three-day program and the more difficult month-long sugar detox. What's more, with the two-week plan you will have both a week to deal with the withdrawals, and a week to enjoy the benefits of a sugarless diet. Once you have exhausted the two weeks, the results will help you decide if a long-term sugar-free lifestyle is for you or not. At least you'll know what life is like on both sides of the fence. The shorter three-day detox is great because you can easily fit it inside of a long weekend. Unfortunately, three days is just long enough to experience the withdrawal symptoms without knowing what it's like once you're past them. On the other hand, a one-month strategy would give you the best under-standing of life without sugar, but a month is really daunting when just starting out.

But again, just because I recommend two weeks doesn't mean that's the best option for you and your body. Pick a length you can stick with and do it. If three days feel more manageable, run with that and don't look back. It's far better to get started with a shorter detox than to plan for a long one and fall through.

## KEY POINTS

In this chapter, we discussed what a zero sugar detox entails.

- A zero sugar detox involves you doing away with all forms of sugar in your diet. This includes alternate sources of sugar such as carbs.
- The plan can last anywhere from three days to 1-2 weeks, a month, or more. Your best option is dependent on what you can handle, so you need to consider your personal situation and diet carefully. I would recommend that you go for the two-week detox, as this will give you the most benefits without jumping into something intimidating like a month-long strategy.

When you are done, the outcome can help determine if you want to continue with the zero sugar lifestyle.

- Because of the addictive nature of sugar, I highly suggest you go cold turkey and embrace the withdrawal headfirst.

Next, we will talk about what these withdrawals will entail and what the detox experience is like.

# WHAT TO EXPECT DURING YOUR DETOX

I wish I could tell you that your upcoming sugar detox will be a breeze, but that is hardly ever the case. Leaving sugar behind is like trying to leave a gang, and there are consequences for abandoning the sugar gang. They come in the form of withdrawal symptoms.

This chapter will lay out the different stages you most likely will experience during your detox journey, and what sort of withdrawal symptoms to expect. Fear not, it's not all doom and gloom. I'll also give you some very practical tips to help you lessen the effects of those symptoms.

**Motivation Stage**

Often when you want to achieve a particular goal, you begin with a powerful feeling of motivation. For instance, take someone who has a goal of getting fit. The first few days are when the motivation is high, and the person goes all out, hitting the gym like never before.

This is usually the first day of your detox when you're excited about the journey you're on to freeing yourself of sugar.

**Powerful Cravings Stage**

Like we talked about earlier, sugar is very addictive, and most people usually consume it in large portions every day. This means you will probably have to deal with cravings, which come right after your initial rush has started to wane.

After you have taken out sugar from your diet, you need to expect to deal with cravings frequently. The intensity of these cravings may differ for each individual. But when you get to this stage, your best option is to replace it with activities that can offer a positive distraction. If you fail to do this, you will spend much of your time thinking about your cravings, and before you know it you may find yourself giving in.

(You'll discover tons of craving busting options in Chapter 9.)

**Withdrawal Stage**

Next comes the Withdrawal Stage. It is at this stage that you can expect to experience a variety of mental, physical and social symptoms.

The symptoms you deal with are dependent on the amount of sugar you have grown accustomed to consuming. The withdrawal symptoms can last from two days to as long as two weeks. The longer you are able to survive without sugar, the less intense your symptoms will become.

You may notice that some symptoms are heightened during specific parts of the day, like between meals. What's more, stress is known to trigger sugar cravings, so you may observe that you experience worse symptoms when you are dealing with stress.

**Mental Symptoms**

A sugar detox can result in numerous mental and emotional symptoms, including:

- **Anxiety:** This may also come with feelings of irritability, restlessness, and nervousness.

You may feel like you are more on edge than normal and have less patience.

- **Depression:** A very common symptom of sugar withdrawal is depression. This comes alongside low mood swings.
- **Change in sleep patterns:** Some individuals may deal with changes in their patterns of sleeping when on a sugar detox. You may also have disrupted sleep and find it difficult to go to sleep at night.
- **Cravings:** In addition to craving sugar, you may observe that you are craving other meals containing carbohydrates like pasta and bread.
- **Problems with concentration:** When you give up sugar, you may deal with concentration issues or "brain fog." It may be impossible to pay attention to tasks at hand, like work or school.

**Physical Symptoms**

One of the most prominent and common physical symptoms of the sugar detox is a headache. In most cases, the headaches come soon after the cravings stage, but it varies between different individuals. Unfortunately, pushing through the headaches is the only way you can get past this stage. Additionally, make sure you are staying hydrated, as this can alleviate a lot of headache symptoms. Think of it as a rite of passage for getting past the addiction to sugar.

These headaches often also accompany a feeling of being physically drained. There are other likely physical symptoms, ranging from fatigue to nausea and dizziness, that you should be aware of.

**Social Symptoms**

As you go through the different stages of the sugar detox process, you need to understand that your life may be affected in other ways that people don't tell you about. One of those major areas is your social life. Below are a few areas that can be impacted.

- **Going out with friends becomes hard:** It can get tricky when you're out with friends for your usual Friday happy hour, and instead of actually ordering a drink you request water. If you have friends who understand, this should not be a problem. Still, it can make hanging out complex since nobody wants to be the unexpected killjoy.
- **Your meal options become limited:** When

out on a date, at a party, or grabbing a bite, your eating options are most likely going to be carb-loaded sugar bombs. You should be prepared to have limited options when you're out. Pro tip: you may want to keep some snacks close, so you don't fall into temptation. If it is a potluck, where all the guests bring their own dish, you're in luck. You can bring a delicious sugar-free recipe that everyone can enjoy.

## End of Symptoms

The prior two stages are typically the most uncomfortable. However, the instant you can make it through those stages, things will become much better.

When you reach this stage, you will feel free, energized, and even able to see life from a new perspective. It will seem like a veil has been lifted from your eyes, and you will have a new outlook on your appearance, health, and life. This last stage is where you will feel the greatest.

## DEALING WITH THE SYMPTOMS OF A SUGAR DETOX

Now that you have learned about many of the stages and symptoms of sugar withdrawal, the next step is to determine the best methods and strategies to help you get past them. Let's take a look at some of these strategies below.

**1. Keep Healthy Snacks Close At All Times**

The reality is that your most tempting cravings will arise when you are close to a donut shop, bakery, restaurant, or other locations offering foods with added sugar. For this reason, you need to be ready. You can do this by getting a lot of healthy snacks and keeping them close.

Stash plenty of these in your car, office desk, laptop bag, or anywhere else you spend a great deal of your time. Purchase portable, non-refrigerated treats like nuts, beef jerky, cheese sticks, etc. All of these will ensure you have something close by when temptation arises.

(We'll talk more about sugar-free snacks options in Chapter 7.)

## 2. Get Rid of All the Sugar in Your Home

Of course, it will be more difficult to stay focused and motivated when the item you are trying to stay away from is staring right at you. For this reason, you will have to clear out all of the sugary items in your home. Since sugar can be hidden even in the most unlikely meals, you will want to take your time to read the labels of all the food products in your home. Doing this will help ensure that you can eradicate all of the frozen, canned, and even packaged meals that have added sugar in them. Or even easier, simply get rid of all your frozen and packaged meals altogether.

## 3. Enhance Your Dietary Fiber

Eating meals with high fiber can aid you in dealing with hunger. This is because it helps keep your blood sugar under control, and helps you deal with side effects like nausea and headaches. Fiber does all of this while also keeping hunger away. Ideal options include legumes, beans, and vegetables, which are all high in fiber.

(We'll talk more about healthy whole food options in Chapter 7.)

## 4. Stay Hydrated

When you increase your fiber intake, it is essential to stay hydrated. This is because more fiber could result in constipation, and drinking more water can help make certain that your stool can easily move out of your system.

What's more, it's easy to confuse dehydration with hunger. So by drinking more water, you can better overcome the urge to eat in excess and keep your cravings in check.

## 5. Stay Away from Artificial Sweeteners

It may seem like a great option to use artificial sweeteners as an alternative when you give up sugar. However, doing this can make you lose sight of your objectives. Studies have shown that artificial sweeteners can encourage sugar dependence and cravings just as badly as the real thing. Artificial sweeteners can also trigger an inflammatory cycle, as well as increase insulin levels. To eradicate sugar from your diet completely, you need to stay away from every kind of sweet food, including those that claim to be sugar-free.

## 6. Exercise

Working out offers numerous benefits when you are on a sugar detox plan. It helps you reduce stress and enhances your energy, both of which can aid you in dealing with withdrawal symptoms like stress-induced cravings and low energy levels.

Plus, exercising will help you burn through your glycogen reserves faster, so that you can start tapping into burning your fat storage sooner. What's more, working out helps you release those beneficial feel-good endorphins.

But a word of caution when it comes to exercise. Don't just decide to jump into a sugar detox and start flipping tractor tires. Stick to an exercise that fits within your current level of physical activity.

### 7. Sleep More

Not getting adequate sleep can make sugar detox symptoms like cravings, fatigue, and depression worse. Also, inadequate sleep has been proven to enhance cravings for sugar and other unhealthy meals, which we talked about in Chapter 3.

Getting adequate sleep has been associated with reduced stress, increased levels of energy, better food choices, and enhanced memory and concentration. All of the things you could use more of during your detox.

## 8. Forgive Yourself

It's not easy to give up all sources of sugar, considering it is something you probably haven't gone a day without in a long time. So if you stray away from your path, don't punish yourself. If you give in, start anew. Don't dwell on it as a failure. Instead, see it as an experience you can learn from to ensure you don't make the same mistake again. For example, if there are specific locations that trigger the most temptation, try to stay away from those areas, or be prepared with snacks and water to get you past it.

## What People Don't Tell You about A Sugar Detox

Even though going on a no sugar-detox plan is going to be beneficial in the long run, you need to know that it is not a comfortable journey. It's very easy to ignore the hard parts and focus only on the good, but it's a journey that requires commitment. You will need to let go of some of those things you have become accustomed to, at least for a short while.

Sugar detox takes time; and with some patience, commitment, and preparation, it will be possible to get through a sugar detox without any critical symptoms. In the end, you will feel better than you ever have.

Don't forget that any symptoms you deal with are not permanent. The symptoms will end, and the benefits you gain will be well worth it.

Like I said at the beginning of the book, if at any point you start to worry that this seems too hard, go to the bonus chapter in the back of the book. I've got a free gift that will make this whole detox thing way easier.

## KEY POINTS

It's good to remember that…

- You will deal with withdrawal symptoms, and this is something that you can't avoid. The reality is that it gets uncomfortable before you start to enjoy all of the benefits. You've heard the saying "It gets worse before it gets better!"
- You are going to experience both physical and mental withdrawal symptoms when you go into the sugar detox plan, so you have to be prepared for it.

- Some of the mental symptoms you will experience include anxiety, depression, changes in sleep patterns, and concentration problems, while the physical symptoms may include headaches, fatigue, and dizziness. However, your goal is to get past these symptoms. Things will become much easier soon after.

When the sugar withdrawal symptoms come, there are ways to deal with it, including:

- Have sugar-free snacks on you at all times
- Drink lots of water, as it's easy to confuse thirst for hunger
- Work out often, so you get those feel-good endorphins going
- Get more sleep
- You have to be prepared for the difficulties that go with a sugar detox. You are going to be making a change to your lifestyle, which means some of your routines may also change. Your social life may take a hit, and it might become challenging to hang out with friends or go on dates due to your limited diet. That said, it's only for the length of the

detox, and the rewards that come with getting sugar out of your life are worth every inconvenience.

And speaking of inconveniences, the next chapter is going to walk you through exactly what you need to stay away from to make your detox a successful one.

# FOODS THAT WILL RUIN YOUR DETOX THE MOMENT YOU EAT THEM

## First, A Reminder: It Will All Be Worth It.

Remember, your goal is to rid your body of sugar and live a healthier life. The following list of foods you'll need to eliminate can be depressing, but letting go of all of these foods is extremely vital.

Anytime you find yourself straying, ask yourself: Would you rather enjoy the fleeting immediate pleasures that come with consuming sugar, or aim for the long-term rewards that come with permanently ridding sugar from your life? If you're reading this book, I'm sure the latter is your objective.

There are tons of foods with sugar that you need to stay away from if you want your sugar detox program to be a success. This is where many people get it wrong, since some food items can be deceiving.

You can read this entire chapter to gain a deep understanding of everything you need to remove from your diet to stick to your detox. You can learn all 61 (yes, 61!) names that sugar goes by. You can also meticulously study every food label at the grocery store.

Or...you can save yourself a lot of time and trouble by simply avoiding anything that comes packaged or in a box, and avoiding carbs. That alone will cut out 95 percent of the foods to avoid.

If you are gung-ho about learning more about everything you should avoid, jump right in!

## HIGH GLYCEMIC/INSULIN INDEX FOODS

Ideally, you want to stay away from high glycemic/insulin index foods. To help make this process less difficult, let's take a detailed look at what the glycemic and insulin indexes are.

**What Is the Glycemic Index?**

The Glycemic Index (GI) is a measurement that lets you know the speed at which your body transforms the carbohydrates in foods into glucose. It is possible for foods with the same level of carbohydrates to have varying GI numbers.

The lower the number, the lower the effect a food item has on your blood sugar. It is usually categorized in the following way:

- Meals with 55 or less = Low (good)
- Meals with 56 - 69 = Medium (reasonable)
- Meals with 70 or higher = High (bad)

If you are consuming packaged meals, you can sometimes find the GI number on the labels, but not usually. However, there are tons of GI lists on the internet for many of the popular foods we consume.

In most cases, whole foods are more likely to have a lower GI as opposed to their processed and refined counterparts.

**Glycemic Index Can Change Based on the Circumstances**

There are a variety of factors that can change the

Glycemic Index number from what you started with to what ends up on your plate. Some of these include:

- **Level of ripeness:** Some fruits gain a higher GI as they ripen. A fantastic example of this is a banana. An unripe banana may come with a GI of 29, while a ripe banana may have a GI of 48.
- **How you prepare your food:** Acid, fiber, and fat tend to reduce the GI number. This is because they reduce the speed of digestion and how quickly the stomach empties. In essence, adding them to your meals will lead to a lower GI. In addition, meals you have prepared and allowed to cool down can have a lower GI when consumed cold, as opposed to when they're still hot. An example of this is a potato. What's more, the longer you prepare starches like rice and pasta, the higher the GI becomes.
- **Food combination:** The kinds of food you eat simultaneously can lower the total GI of a meal. This is possible if you combine foods with a low GI to those with high ones, or add proteins and/or healthy oils.

The speed at which you digest meals, along with your age, can have an impact on the way your body deals with carbs. The size of a meal portion is also significant, as the higher the number of carbs you consume, the more impact they will have on your blood sugar.

However, just because a food item does not have a high GI does not mean it is exceptionally healthy. Again, whole fresh foods are your best bets, combined with a low glycemic load. You want to stay away from meals that have a high glycemic load during your sugar detox, and in general.

**What Is the Insulin Index?**

A food's Insulin Index (II) shows how much the item enhances the insulin concentration in your blood two hours after you've consumed a meal. This shares some similarities to the Glycemic Index; however, it focuses on your blood insulin levels instead of your blood glucose levels.

The II signifies an assessment of meal portions with their total caloric content. The II is also vital because there are meals that can trigger an insulin response in your body, even when there are no carbs in the meal. Furthermore, some meals result in an insulin response that is not proportionate to their carbohydrate load.

The insulin and glucose scores of many meals usually correlate, but bakery products and meals high in protein can trigger responses that are more than their glycemic counterparts.

**Apps That Help You Find a Food's Index**

Since calculating your food index yourself can be tedious, there are apps that can help you out. You can install them on your computer and/or smartphone and utilize them in getting accurate scores for your meals.

Some great apps you can use include:

- **Glycemic Index, Load Net Carbs:** This app gives you the chance to search and see the Glycemic Index and GI load for various kinds of foods. It is easy to use and extremely convenient.
- **Glyx: Glycemic Load & Index:** This is another excellent app that you can install on Android and iOS devices. It is a very portable guide that offers you the GI of various common meals.

- **The Low-Glycal Diet™ by BioFit:** Unlike the other options, this outlines a low GI diet to follow. It is based on the most recent medical research.
- **DiaLife:** Want something to help you monitor your GI? Then this is the app to use. It comes with a calculator that helps you instantly calculate the GI in meals, the number of carbohydrates, lipids, and more.
- **Glycemic Index of Products:** Here, you get a product list alongside the GI number of each of them. It is a great app to download if you want assistance with your sugar detox.

In addition to the above, some apps can help you calculate your Insulin Index. These include:

- **SiDiary6**
- **dbees.com**

**Foods to Avoid**

The list of foods in this category can be slightly heart-wrenching, but *you need to think about the benefits of avoiding these meals as opposed to thinking about how much you are going to miss them*. Again, remember that this is mostly temporary. Once you're done with your sugar detox, these foods can be saved for special treats. That being said, let's take a look at some foods to avoid.

**Anything That Includes Added Sugar**

This is a no-brainer. You will need to forgo any food that contains added sugar. This includes:

- Ice Cream
- Sodas
- Gelato
- Frozen Yogurt
- Custard
- Rice Pudding
- Cookies
- Cereal
- Candies

This also includes those food items categorized as "healthy" sugar. Since our bodies categorize all sugar the same way, the effects are usually the same. So, it doesn't really matter. You will still need to let them go. Good examples include:

- Honey
- Greek Yogurt

- Granola
- Ketchup

**White Flour**

When you strip the bran and germ from a grain of wheat, like what happens during the creation of white flour, you are left with only carbohydrates, which your body absorbs very quickly. This fast absorption comes with the urge to consume more. This is because you won't feel as full as you would have if you had eaten a meal with the protein and fiber of the entire (or "whole") grain.

Also, a type of carbohydrate in wheat known as amylopectin A is more potent in white flour. This is because the absence of fiber ensures that it is converted into blood sugar with less difficulty, as opposed to other forms of carbohydrates.

As you can imagine, the glycemic load of white flour is extremely high, which means it should not be present in your diet. The modern white flour we consume today also comes with a protein known as gliadin, which triggers the brain's feel-good effect, which is why common white flour foods like pasta, bread and crackers are often known as "comfort" food.

The bottom line is that you need to stay away from meals that are made from refined white flour. Examples of foods in this category include:

- Doughnuts
- Bread
- Cakes
- Chips
- Crackers
- Pretzels
- Pasta
- Cookies
- Cereals
- Muffins
- Pizza Crust
- Pie Crust

The above are only a few meals made from white flour. If you observe the list above closely, you will notice that a majority of the meals that have white flour are junk food. In addition to white flour, these foods also often come with added sugar and other damaging ingredients like preservatives and artificial colors.

**White Rice**

You may believe that white rice doesn't pose any threat. But the truth is that it is just like eating sugar in a bowl. It goes through a refining process very similar to white flour, one that transforms the whole rice grain into fiberless starch.

The GI of rice varies depending on the kind of rice and how long you spend cooking it. However, all kinds of rice will result in a sugar spike when you consume it. Worse still, we tend to consume starchy food in larger portions, because it doesn't make us feel as full. This is because of the absent fiber content, which would have slowed the digestion of these meals.

According to recent studies, consuming white rice can lead to a drastic increase in your blood sugar. This takes place especially when you eat it frequently or in large amounts.

**Processed/Packaged Foods**

Many people love processed and packaged foods since they are convenient options for cooking meals at home. However, these foods are often packed with a huge amount of sugar content that can send your body spiking into a sugar overdose. Also, many of these processed foods consist of refined white carbs, which as we've seen is a big no-no for your zero sugar detox.

The most common include:

- Microwave Popcorn
- Granola Bars
- Flavored Nuts
- Instant Ramen
- Margarine
- Cereal
- Most frozen dinners

## All Grains (But Especially Refined Grains)

Grains are hard, small, and edible dry seeds which you can find on grass-like plants known as cereals. In many countries, they're very popular since they offer a higher amount of energy than any other food group.

They can be consumed by humans and can also be used for livestock, which makes them extremely crucial to every economy. However, during your sugar detox, you will have to stay away from grains, including the good ones.

Whole grains are healthy and nutritious, but they

still contain a good amount of starch to spike your body's blood sugar. But even worse are the refined grains, which are similar to whole grains except that all the nutritious parts have been stripped out, through a chemical process known as "bleaching." The only thing left after the refining process is high-calorie and high-carb starch, which makes the effect on your body even worse. This is the refined grain family (white flour, white rice) that we talked about earlier.

Other examples of grains include:

- Oats
- Barley
- Millet
- Triticale
- Wild Rice
- Corn
- Quinoa
- Buckwheat

There are instances where products made from grains are included in processed meals too. Look at the labels to determine meals with any type of grains, and stay away from them during your sugar detox.

**Starchy Vegetables**

Contrary to popular belief, not all vegetables are healthy for you. Some veggies are just a bowl of starch in disguise. They have a high GI, which you now know can lead to a blood sugar spike.

Although these veggies offer you some benefits nutrition-wise, you will need to avoid them if you want to get the best results from your sugar detox plan. There are many veggies in this category, and some of the common ones include:

- Butternut Squash
- Acorn Squash
- Pumpkins
- Potatoes
- Sweet Potatoes/Yams
- Taro
- Parsnips
- Corn
- Green Peas

**Dried Fruit**

The goal of drying fruit is to ensure it is portable and able to last longer. This is ideal if you are out camping or hiking and need something to provide you with instant energy.

However, even with the benefits, there are still a few major drawbacks. Dried fruit goes through a process that removes the water, which makes the fruit more condensed than it originally was. In addition, many dried fruits come with added sugar, which tends to spike your blood sugar even faster.

Many dry fruits have so much sugar that they outweigh the benefits they provide. Even though they are not as unhealthy as eating a candy bar, they should not be your go-to snack during a detox.

## Juice

If the goal is to spike your blood sugar quickly, a glass of fruit juice is the ideal option. It consists almost entirely of pure sugar, with no fiber or protein to get in the way of being instantly absorbed.

Vegetable juices are a seemingly healthier option, but they should be avoided as well. During the production of these juices, a whole lot of fruit is added to give them a sweeter taste, which means they are not ideal for your detox either.

Even those commercial juice brands that claim that the amount of sugar in them is low can still trigger a sugar rush. Instead, drink flavored water if you really must have something with added flavor. Better yet, add some slices of lemon or cucumber to your water. It's rejuvenating and hydrating, and doesn't consist of any added sugar.

**Sodas**

Sodas are cartoonishly easy in the modern American diet to get a hold of almost for free, and so this tends to be the main source of added sugar for most people. They usually come in regular and diet variants, but you will need to stay away from both during your sugar detox.

First, regular soda is literally liquid sugar mixed with water, various chemicals, and coloring. They do not offer even a single nutritional benefit, and should not be a part of any healthy diet, especially a sugar detox.

As far as sugar substitutes, it's true that there's no evidence that they raise either blood sugar or insulin levels. The issue is that when we eat something that tastes sweet, whether from real or artificial sugar, we are more likely to turn to something else that's sweet, which in most cases will be loaded with real sugar. And when we don't, we suffer from the same powerful cravings we discussed earlier.

For the sake of the detox, it's best to rid anything that tastes super-sweet from your diet.

**Sugar Goes By Many Names**

Stay away from any food that comes with syrup or sugar and you will get the best results from your detox. However, as you must know by now, sugar comes in a ton of different forms and is known by nearly a hundred different names. Do yourself a favor and learn every one of them.

Below are a few of the most common names for sugar:

**Basic Simple Sugars**

- Lactose
- Dextrose
- Fructose
- Glucose
- Maltose
- Galactose
- Sucrose

**Granulated or Solid Sugars**

- Beet Sugar
- Cane Juice Crystals
- Castor Sugar
- Crystalline Fructose
- Cane Sugar
- Powdered Sugar
- Brown Sugar
- Table or Granulated Sugar
- Corn Syrup Solids
- Demerara Sugar
- Diastatic Malt
- Florida Crystals
- Ethyl Maltol
- Glucose Syrup Solids
- Muscovado Sugar
- Golden Sugar
- Panela Sugar
- Maltodextrin
- Grape Sugar
- Raw Sugar
- Icing Sugar
- Sucanat
- Date Sugar
- Turbinado Sugar
- Dextrin
- Coconut Sugar

- Yellow Sugar

## Syrup or Liquid Sugars

- Agave Nectar/Syrup
- Blackstrap Molasses
- Brown Rice Syrup
- Carob Syrup
- Evaporated Cane Juice
- Buttered Sugar/Buttercream
- Golden Syrup
- Corn Syrup
- Fruit Juice Concentrate
- Malt Syrup
- Maple Syrup
- Invert Sugar
- High-Fructose Corn Syrup (HFCS)
- Honey
- Caramel
- Refiner's Syrup
- Barley Malt
- Fruit Juice
- Molasses
- Rice Syrup
- Sorghum Syrup
- Treacle

## KEY POINTS

There are many things you will be unable to eat during a sugar detox diet. One of the most important are foods that have a high Glycemic/Insulin Index load.

The Glycemic Index is a number that teaches you how fast your body transforms the carbohydrates in any food you consume to glucose. The following are a few ways to determine if a food item is good or bad using their GI score:

- Meals with 55 or less = Low (good)
- Meals with 56 - 69 = Medium (reasonable)
- Meals with 70 or higher = High (bad)

You will need to stay away from numerous foods like:

- Sodas
- Grains
- Some fruits
- Processed/packaged meals
- Starchy veggies
- Dried fruits
- Sweetened dairy products

- Artificial sweeteners
- Condiments
- Everything that contains added sugar
- You may need to go through the labels to determine the ingredients in any product you are about to consume, to ensure there is no sugar. Better still, just stop eating anything that comes in a package or box. That alone will take the majority of the guesswork out of what you can't have for the duration of your detox.

Now that you know which meals to avoid, in the next chapter we'll take a look at foods that you can eat and enjoy.

# WHAT TO EAT TO CRUSH YOUR DETOX FROM DAY 1

S ince most processed foods consist of sugar in hidden forms, your list of meals to eat is limited. However, this does not mean you don't have great options available. In this chapter, we will cover examples of the things you can eat during the sugar detox process. Let's take a look at them in more detail.

## Non-Starchy Vegetables

When it comes to a sugar detox, one type of food that should constitute a major part of your meals are vegetables. In fact, your vegetable options are almost limitless, and many have little to no effect on your blood-sugar level. They even offer you tons of minerals, vitamins, fiber, and antioxidants, all of which are healthy for you.

So anytime you are confused as to what to eat, remember that the vast majority of veggies are your friend. Even if you avoid the starchy vegetables we covered in the previous chapter, you will still be left with many options. They include:

**Cruciferous Vegetables**

Many vegetables like cauliflower, broccoli, and cabbage are in the cruciferous family. They come filled with cancer-battling properties and have the least number of calories and sugar. What's more, these vegetables aid with the repair and growth of tissues in the body. They can also help protect your body from sun damage, which can result in premature aging.

On top of the ones already mentioned, other examples of cruciferous vegetables include:

- Kale
- Watercress
- Bok Choy
- Brussels Sprouts
- Collard Greens

- Arugula
- Radishes

**Green, Leafy and Fibrous Vegetables**

Green, leafy, and fibrous vegetables offer tons of nutrition and fiber. They are amazing options for a no-sugar diet. However, if you were not already a fan of these vegetables before your sugar detox, it might take some time for your stomach to adapt. This is because they can affect your gastrointestinal tract. So, make sure to drink enough fluids to avoid constipation.

Some examples of these kinds of vegetables include:

- Cucumbers
- Celery
- White Mushrooms
- Spinach
- Bell Peppers
- Asparagus
- Tomatoes
- Lettuce

**Proteins**

The fact that you are on a no-sugar diet doesn't

mean you can't take in protein. In fact, protein is crucial to your sugar detox, as it helps in keeping you full and feeling satisfied. One of the most important functions of protein in your diet is that it can reduce cravings, appetite and hunger levels, while also helping to boost metabolism. Below are the most common options.

**Lean Red Meats**

All lean red meats are ideal for a sugar detox. This is because they have no sugar content whatsoever, and they are a great source of saturated fat. Good examples include:

- Round Cuts
- Choice or Select Cuts
- Brisket
- Flank Steak
- Pot Roast
- Top Sirloin
- T-Bone
- Tenderloin and Other Loin Cuts
- Lean game, such as bison, venison, pheasant and duck

**Poultry and Pork**

Turkey, chicken, and pork are great lean protein sources, which make them ideal to include in a sugar detox. As a source of high amounts of protein, even when consumed alongside starch, they can help slow down the speed at which your meals are absorbed in your body.

**Seafood**

Seafood also makes an excellent protein source. It doesn't affect your blood sugar as much as other foods when consumed, and specific types of fish contain high amounts of essential fatty acids, things that the body needs to stay in great shape but is unable to produce itself.

Essential Omega-3 fatty acids, like the ones found in fish and seafood, also have the capacity to avert insulin resistance. They do this by enhancing the sensitivity of your cells to insulin. What's more, they help in building your skin's natural moisturizers and ensure your skin stays hydrated. Fish and shellfish have also long been known to offer cardiovascular protection and benefits. The best examples for a zero sugar detox include:

- Salmon
- Trout

- Oysters
- Mackerel
- Herring
- Anchovies
- Sardines
- Crab
- Scallops

**Healthy Fats**

If you remember from the previous chapters, it's not necessarily fat consumption that makes you fat. It's sugar that is restoring your glycogen reserves, preventing you from ever using your fat storage as fuel.

Since you won't be getting the majority of your calories from carbs, you'll need to adjust your diet to add in more healthy fat to get your daily caloric needs.

Examples of healthy fats include:

- Avocado
- Cheese
- Olive Oil
- Dark Chocolate
- Butter (yes, butter!)
- Eggs

- Fatty Fish
- Chia Seeds
- Coconut/Coconut Oil

**Green Tea**

The benefits provided by green tea are well-known. This is because it's very rich in antioxidants known as flavonoids. The flavonoids you find in green tea are called catechins, and they are extremely powerful in ensuring there is no oxidative damage to cells. This antioxidant is even more potent than Vitamin C and E in performing this role.

Also, green tea is naturally free of calories. This benefit, alongside all of the other benefits it offers, makes it an amazing addition to your sugar detox.

**Legumes and Nuts**

Nuts and legumes offer extraordinary health benefits to the body. They are a great protein source, especially for vegetarians, as they consist of a high amount of fiber and are not difficult to prepare. They are also great choices to be used as snacks during a sugar detox.

**Legumes** can help in the management and reduction of your sugar levels. This is because they are high in fiber content. Lentils especially are filled with both insoluble and soluble dietary fiber. The soluble fiber aids in slowing down the absorption of sugar molecules. The body does not see the insoluble fiber as sugar or carbohydrates, and it goes through the digestive tract seamlessly.

The fiber you find in legumes aids in slowing down the entire digestive process. This ensures that you stay full for a longer time, and helps to stabilize your blood sugar and insulin levels.

On top of all forms of beans, lentils and peas (including chickpeas), a particularly great legume for people on a zero sugar detox is soybeans, because they're so versatile. You can eat them roasted as a snack on the go, cooked as a side for dinner (known in that form as edamame), or prepared as a stand-alone dish like tempeh or tofu.

**Water, Water, Water**

Water is extremely crucial in any healthy lifestyle, and it is even more crucial during your sugar detox. Drinking water helps with digestion and improves your hydration. Water is also ideal for your overall well-being and health. Stay hydrated, people!

**Herbs and Spices**

During your sugar detox, herbs and spices will quickly become your best friends. They are not just a great means of adding tons of flavor to your meals without the inclusion of any sugar, sodium, or additional calories, but they have health benefits too.

Numerous studies have proven that specific spices and herbs can positively affect blood sugar levels, lower inflammation, and slow the glycation process, which as we discussed in an earlier chapter results in your skin looking more wrinkled and older than it really is.

Some specific spices like allspice, cinnamon, and ginger are most effective against glycation. Also, herbs like rosemary and tarragon were observed to be efficient in the prevention of glycation.

Common examples of herbs and spices that are typically easy to find in grocery stores include:

- Garlic
- Parsley
- White or Black Pepper
- Basil
- Red Pepper Flakes
- Mint
- Rosemary

- Oregano
- Dill Weed
- Saffron
- Sage
- Cayenne Pepper
- Thyme
- Paprika
- Cilantro

Two common spices, however, are so extraordinarily good for you, they deserve a closer look.

**Cinnamon**

Cinnamon is a very common spice in the sugar detox plan because it can aid the body in becoming more sensitive to insulin. Basically, it urges the cells to notice the insulin in the body and work to eradicate sugar in the correct manner.

**Turmeric**

Turmeric is another well-known spice that is commonly used in Indian cuisines and is what gives yellow curry its beautiful color. Turmeric has been proven to offer numerous benefits to your health, as it can avert carcinogens from being produced when used with fried and barbecued meats. It also consists of elements that have been shown to restrict cancer progression in the body.

Herbs and spices can also be great when infused as a tea. There are numerous tea brands that have amazing benefits and have already done the hard work for you of mixing the spices in a pleasing ratio. The great news is that you can consume as much tea as you want during your sugar detox.

## HOW TO EAT AT EACH MEAL

The main objective of a sugar detox plan is to alter how you eat so that you're naturally consuming meals that are more nutritious, delicious, and sugar-free. Once you have adopted these new eating habits, you will feel full longer, and won't experience those midday sugar crashes. What's more, your cravings for sugar will start to vanish.

A great way to start your zero sugar detox meal plan is to make simple choices from the following list.

### Pick a Protein

Protein, regardless of where it comes from, is extremely satisfying. It can make you feel full and ensure you consume fewer overall calories during the meal. In addition, beginning every meal with a source of protein ensures that you don't experience any sugar spikes. Instead, your body channels all of its resources into transforming that protein into amino acids, which help your body control blood-sugar levels. Pick one of the numerous sources of protein mentioned previously, and include it in your meal.

**Pick a Fat**

Eating the right type of fat alongside your meals can avert spikes in your blood sugar as well. So, when whipping up your meal during the sugar detox, don't forget to include healthy fats in whatever you are consuming. More of your daily calories will come from fats now that you've taken carbs out of your diet.

**Pick a Vegetable (Or Two)**

Of course, you want to make sure you include a veggie or two in your meals. Like we discussed earlier, they are nutritious and don't have a negative impact on your blood sugar. Observe your meals and include your best vegetable options using the list provided.

**Don't Forget to Add Herbs and Spices**

Like we discussed earlier, preparing your meals with herbs and spices is a great way to give it a delicious flavor. While eating veggies, you can include them to make it less bland. Take a look at the herbs and spices we covered, and pick your favorites from those listed.

## WHAT TO DO RIGHT NOW

To ensure the best chance of success in your detox, here are a few initial things to do before anything else.

### Purge Your Kitchen

You will want to get rid of all food in your kitchen that does not align with the criteria we've discussed. Read those labels and get rid of anything containing sugar. Better still, remove all of the packaged and processed meals in your house, since we know how unhealthy they can be for you. If you have condiments, you may want to get rid of those as well. You have to be truthful and honest with yourself when doing this, as this is the only way you are going to get the best results.

### Make A Meal Plan

Determine the meals you will make for the week and put a shopping list together. This will help you stay focused on purchasing only healthy options once you're at the store.

**Restock Your Snack Pile**

When you start to deal with sugar cravings, which you inevitably will, having healthy snacks on hand can be your saving grace. Go shopping and restock your fridge with things like nuts, celery, cucumbers, carrots, roasted soybeans, beef jerky, and high-quality cheese. Separate them into individual plastic bags, so that you immediately have a snack to take with you each time you leave the house.

From all we have listed, you will still have numerous meals and food options to choose from even after eliminating those with sugar. They may not be the same as you are used to, but they are nutritious and healthier for your body, and soon your body will crave healthy foods instead of sugar.

KEY POINTS

Your meal options will have to change in order for the sugar detox plan to be successful.

Some of the best choices available to you include:

- **Protein:** like poultry, beans, pork, meat, and even seafood. They do not consist of sugar and are essential for your body to function at peak capacity. However, if you are going to be consuming any animal, you want to make sure they were raised with natural food and not artificial supplements.
- **Fats:** Healthy fats are an essential part of any diet, including your no-sugar diet. It does not have any impact on your blood sugar levels and is vital for your body's peak performance.
- **Vegetables:** Your vegetable options are almost limitless (minus the starchy variety), and many have little to no effect on your blood-sugar level. They offer you tons of minerals, vitamins, fiber, and antioxidants, all of which are great for your overall health.
- Other things to consume as much as you want include legumes, nuts, and green tea, plus of course plenty of water. Lastly, herbs and spices are a great addition to help your meals feel less bland and add flavor, or in tea form for a delicious pick-me-up.

To ensure you are eating the right way during your mealtimes, make certain you do the following:

- Keep your meals simple
- Pick a protein
- Pick a fat
- Pick a vegetable or two
- Add some herbs and spices

You want your sugar detox plan to go as seamlessly as possible. For this reason, you will want to do the following:

- Purge your kitchen
- Make a meal list
- Restock your fridge with new, healthier snacks

With those steps complete, your sugar detox is well underway. However, there is still one more crucial piece that needs to be in place in order to make this the biggest success it can be. The next chapter is going to help you put this last piece of the puzzle in place. Ignore at your own peril!

## THE MOST CRUCIAL STEP: ACCOUNTABILITY

Addiction is something that's not easy to overcome. Since sugar addiction can be especially challenging to deal with, many people begin the sugar detox program and find themselves quickly straying. This is normal, but many people don't understand this and end up blaming themselves, never to continue. Many are so ashamed about their inability to see the goal through to the end that they refuse to seek help from those around them.

But it's very understandable to battle with remaining on track while dealing with your sugar addiction. After all, your mind and body have grown to depend on the excess amount of sugar you have been feeding them. Disrupting all of the mental and physical patterns that you have developed over the years can be difficult. This is where being accountable comes in.

## What Is Accountability, And Why Is It Vital to Your Detox?

There are numerous definitions of this word, but in general terms, being accountable means that you are taking responsibility for your behaviors and actions. However, when it involves a sugar detox, there's a lot more involved. The truth is that to attain all of the benefits that come with sugar detoxing, holding ourselves accountable is one of the most important things we can do.

Sugar detox is a form of recovery, and as we've seen in the earlier chapters, it's not exactly easy. However, to succeed you must face the emotions, behaviors, and situations that you will experience during the detox process. There are numerous ways to stay accountable, but having family members, mentors, and friends in our lives to hold us to our promises can be of great help. This can ensure that you're remaining on the right path and channeling your energy into vital things, which at this point is ridding your body of sugar.

## HOW TO CHOOSE YOUR ACCOUNTABILITY PARTNER

Choosing an accountability partner is solely your choice. It's about you, so you need to pick someone you're comfortable around. This could be a mentor, family member, spouse, senior member of your church or school, and so on. These potential partners can be thought of in the following groups:

- **Those who have experienced the same and won:** These individuals have been able to overcome the particular battle you are presently fighting. Ideally, individuals who have already completed a sugar detox program and excelled should be your first option. This is because they'll understand the struggles involved, and be able to provide you with the motivation and advice you need to be successful as well.
- **Those who care about you:** Since these people will have your best interest at heart, they will be more willing to motivate you to succeed. They will help ensure that your goal becomes a reality with motivation and encouragement.

- **Someone on the same level as you:** If you have a peer who is dealing with the same struggles as you, they can be a great accountability partner. However, this is a trickier option, and you need to be very careful here. If you fail to pick the right person, you may end up with someone who drags you farther away from your goal.

Now that you've learned about the kinds of accountability partners, let's look at a few general rules you can follow that will help you pick the right one.

### Choose Someone You Trust

Ideally, your accountability partner will be someone inherently trustworthy. If your circle of friends includes certain toxic individuals, you may unknowingly end up with someone who will be a detriment to your detox. Go through your coworkers, friends, and loved ones to find the person you will be most comfortable with.

### Choose Someone Who Does Not Judge

Going on a sugar detox can sometimes be a strange concept to people who have no inkling as to what it involves. Even worse is when this kind of person is extremely judgmental. For this reason, you need to find a partner who won't judge you, even if they don't understand the concept. You should feel comfortable telling this person everything you are facing during the process, without any fear that you will be made fun of.

You need to be able to tell your accountability partner everything, or it will make the entire purpose of having one irrelevant. Numerous people make this mistake with physical trainers, and that's why they hardly make any progress. The idea is to go with someone you feel a healthy dynamic with when you share inner fears.

**Choose Someone Who Is Willing to Call You Out**

Conversely, if you have a partner who excessively validates all of your actions, you may never get the push you require to make the change you're after. You can't choose someone who is afraid to call you out when needed. Doing this will defeat the entire purpose. Instead, look for someone willing to gently but firmly bring awareness to your errors; a person who won't be scared of pointing out when you stray away from the path of your detox.

Go with an accountability partner who is flexible

and can support you through the difficult times, while still keeping you to your promise. This kind of person will ensure you stay accountable and focused on your objective.

**Choose Someone Who Knows That It Is Normal to Stray**

Go with a partner who understands that straying away from the path is not a failed end, but instead a normal part of the process. This kind of partner will allow you to learn from your experiences, instead of using them as a form of embarrassment.

## GUIDELINES TO SET WITH YOUR ACCOUNTABILITY PARTNER

In order for your accountability partnership to work, you will need to set a few guidelines up in advance. Most importantly, you need to establish expectations with your selected partner. These expectations should cover communication, how you want to be motivated, and how you can motivate one another if you select with a peer who is also going through a detox.

You can begin by letting them know about your situation. If they seem to understand and sympathize, ask if they can do the following with you:

- Hold you accountable
- Encourage you because you will need it
- Listen to you when you are struggling
- Be willing to help you solve problems when you require assistance
- Understand that if you slip up, you just need some encouragement to keep going

## Respect the Rules

If you both agree that you will communicate on a specific schedule, make sure you follow through. The more you show your partner how serious you are about ridding yourself of sugar, the more seriously they will take you and your goals.

## Share Honestly

Many people who fail at getting over an addiction do so because they never speak up about their problems and struggles. If you find the temptation rising to consume something sweet during your detox, reach out to your partner instantly. Don't hold back until the situation is worse. Speak up on time and speak up frequently. Often it's not that you're craving something sweet, but you're craving an escape from something that's stressing you out. Talk it over with your accountability partner to work it out, before you demolish a family size bag of chips.

**Own Up to Your Mistakes**

If you do not keep a promise you have made at some point, own up to it and don't deflect. Tell your partner the honest reason and be responsible for it.

Don't forget that this person is named an accountability partner for a reason. Even if you do stray from your objectives, the act of being accountable will provide you with more insight as to why you were unable to achieve your goals during this slip. If you choose the right accountability partner, you will develop yourself in many ways, in addition to achieving the goal you've set for yourself.

Lastly, if you succeed, remember to share your success with them. They were with you through the struggle, and it is only right that they are with you when you succeed too.

**Increase Your Accountability Even More**

In addition to getting an accountability partner,

there are a few ways you can make yourself even more accountable.

## Make Your Goals Public

By making your goals public, you leverage all the people around you to keep you accountable. Public accountability is extremely powerful when it involves achieving a goal. As humans, it is easy to doubt ourselves, especially when we're trying to make a huge change in our lives. Anytime you're trying to start something big and intimidating, like a new job, a new business, or a new lifestyle change, your brain will do everything possible to tell you why it's a bad idea. This is the way we are hardwired, so you need to accept it and make plans to combat it. By making your detox goal public and asking for accountability, you give yourself the chance to think more clearly, and to take a giant leap into the new lifestyle you have chosen.

If this is your first time requesting public account-ability, it may seem strange and uncomfortable for you. But this is normal, as it is only your brain fighting your choice once more. Accept these feel-ings and let yourself take this important step. If you stay around people who know you and care about your well-being, the support they offer can help you stay motivated for as long as you need.

**Use Social Media**

If you're an avid user of social media, you can use it to your advantage as well. There are tons of no-sugar diet support groups out there. Search for ones you like and become a member.

There are numerous benefits attached to this, the most important being that you'll meet people who are dealing with the same struggles as you. You will also get the motivation you need, alongside numerous tips and strategies from people in your shoes. What's more, you can also get an accountability partner from groups like these. This way, you'll have someone to regularly reach out to for support, anytime you feel the temptation rising.

KEY POINTS

In this chapter, you've discovered the importance of accountability.

Being accountable is crucial to your sugar detox plan. Accountability means taking responsibility for your actions and ensuring you do everything to complete the goal you have set for yourself.

To stay accountable, there are numerous routes to take, the most important being to find an accountability partner. Ideally, it's best to choose someone neutral but who still cares about your well-being. To choose the right accountability partner, they need to have most, if not all, of the following attributes:

- Someone who does not judge
- Someone who cares about you
- Someone who knows that making mistakes is part of the process
- Someone who is not scared of calling you out when you stray
- An accountability partner could be a friend, colleague or family member. It could also be someone who has gone through what you are going through presently.

Once you finally settle on an accountability partner, you should go through a few initial steps:

- Set up guidelines
- State your expectations
- Go through your goals

- If you would like to add some more pressure to ensure you stick to your detox, you can make your goals public so that everyone around you can keep you in check. You can use social media to join groups and find people who have the same interests as you, or choose more than one accountability partner.

With that said, go find your accountability partner(s) and get started! You are so close to finally jumping right into your zero sugar detox, and I am so freakin' excited for what's in store for you on the other side.

## WHEN CRAVING REARS ITS UGLY FACE

When you are on a sugar detox, you will deal with sugar cravings regularly. This is normal. At some point, your sugar addict brain will rear its ugly face and demand cake! Your brain will kick and scream until it gets what it wants, but all is not lost.

Your brain has been spoiled for far too long, having not felt the sting of rejection. Sugar brain won't know how to handle it at first and will kick and scream even louder because that's its only trick.

Stand strong. You might have sugar on the brain for now, but it won't last forever. Eventually, the kicking and screaming will end as your brain figures out that that doesn't work anymore. An adjustment period is ahead that you both will have to work through together.

The great news is that your brain's sugar craving usually only lasts around five to twenty minutes, depending on the individual. Your objective should be to deal with these cravings without straying. If you can do this, the rest becomes easier.

Let's jump in to see what we can do when our brain throws a sugar craving tantrum.

## DEALING WITH SUGAR CRAVINGS

Knowing the reasons for your sugar cravings is only one piece of the puzzle. However, if you want to get rid of the cravings completely, you will need to change your habits. The following are some of the healthy habits that can help you deal with sugar cravings when they come calling.

**Consume a Healthy Meal**

You need to understand that sugar cravings are different from hunger. Like we stated earlier, a craving is your brain seeking a reward. If this craving comes up when you are also hungry, it can be hard to overcome it.

In fact, when a craving is merged with hunger, the urge can be so powerful as to be almost unstoppable. This is bad for your sugar detox and can place you back to where you started.

If you experience sugar cravings when you are hungry, you may want to eat a healthy meal or snack immediately. Meals with a high amount of protein are one of the best bets for dealing with hunger.

When craving sugar, it can seem frustrating to eat real food. However, if you are serious about your sugar detox and the goals you have put in place, you will realize that all of the efforts will be beneficial in the end, even if it sucks that moment.

**Enjoy a Hot Bath or Shower**

Many people who deal with sugar cravings have observed that taking a hot bath or shower can be rejuvenating and helpful in dealing with them. However, the water needs to be hot, but not so hot that it's uncomfortable.

**Take a Walk**

Taking a brisk walk outside is another thing that can work. If you enjoy running, that's also a great choice. In addition to helping distract you from your craving, it can also release feel-good chemicals in your brain, which can work in getting rid of the cravings.

If it's impossible to go outside, you can do some squats, push-ups, or other forms of light exercise.

## Drink Some Apple Cider Vinegar

Adding one tablespoon of apple cider vinegar to a two-liter bottle of water, then gradually drinking it all day, can aid in minimizing sugar cravings. According to a study written in the *Journal of Functional Foods*, it was proven that ingesting vinegar daily even minimizes the levels of blood sugar in healthy adults who are prone to developing type 2 diabetes.

## Practice Mindfulness

In most instances, sugar cravings are linked with your overall level of stress. This is why mindfulness can offer immense benefits.

Read a book, take a mindful walk, or just relax on your bed to get more peace of mind.

Also, you can try out this guided meditation, which lasts only five minutes, by following the steps below:

- Set a timer on your phone for five minutes.

- Spend the first minute or two focusing on your breathing. You can do this by inhaling and exhaling slowly and deliberately.
- As you go on, observe how your cravings creep up during your meditation. Notice if you're really craving sugar or if you're feeling guilty and stressed. Do you have any emotions associated with cravings?
- More importantly, observe the sensations that these thoughts develop in your body. Notice the things you feel and the areas you feel it. Observe if it makes you uncomfortable to hang on to these feelings and not react.
- Once the timer is up, go back to focusing on your breathing for a minute again. When you are done, you should notice that the cravings have lessened considerably, or perhaps have left altogether.

**Enjoy A Healthy Afternoon Snack**

There are instances when you crave sugar during the day when you need energy. This is even more common if you are a working person trying to do a detox. When this happens, as opposed to falling for the temptation and eating sugar, choose a high protein snack to offer you the energy you need.

**Stay Hydrated**

In order to perform a variety of functions each day, our body requires adequate amounts of water. Water aids in helping us stay energized, enhances elimination and digestion, and provides a host of other functions.

Besides, studies prove that being properly hydrated before you eat a meal can help you feel more satisfied. This averts excess eating and may result in weight loss. When you feel full, you are less likely to deal with sugar cravings.

**Get Adequate Sleep**

Lack of sleep enhances the production of ghrelin, which is a hunger hormone. In one study, participants were limited to only four hours of sleep each night by the researchers. Then, when the scientists showed them pictures of unhealthy and sugary meals, it activated the brain's reward center of the participants. What this implies is that we have a higher possibility of yearning for sugar when actually it is sleep that we're after.

Shoot for a solid eight hours of sleep each night, as this can help you greatly minimize your sugar cravings.

## Drink Some Tea

When the sugar cravings come, reach out for a cup of tea instead. Even before the tea is done steeping, your sugar cravings may have diminished. Plus, the flavor from the tea can help occupy your taste buds.

## Other Helpful Ideas

If none of the above work, there are a few other things that can help you deal with your sugar cravings:

- **Speak to a friend:** Reach out to someone close to you who knows and understands what you're dealing with. Let them know that you're dealing with craving and request some encouragement. This is exactly what your accountability partner is for.
- **Stay away from specific triggers:** Try to stay away from specific locations or activities that can trigger cravings. If you experience cravings when walking past your

favorite restaurant, you may want to avoid it during your detox.

- **Read through your goals:** It can be of great benefit to carry a list of your goals with you and the reasons why you want to rid sugar from your life. This is because remembering things like these off the top of your head can be difficult when you have a sugar craving. Having a list of your goals close-by can help you stay focused when things get tough.

- **Think about the future and the benefits of ridding your system of sugar:** Do you want to lose weight or have more energy? Or perhaps you are after overall happiness? By thinking about the future, you can take your mind off the present where you are dealing with cravings. Besides, thinking about what you want to achieve will help you stay in line even if the sugar cravings do come up.

## Most Importantly, Don't Beat Yourself Up

If you do succumb to your cravings, make certain that you don't beat yourself up. The last thing you need is to believe you have wrecked your entire detox process because you consumed a piece of chocolate. Even though you may have delayed your process, it is not over yet.

You can still transition into the sugar-free life you desire, so long as you are ready to dust yourself off and get back up. Remember that this is part of the process, and all you have to do is pick up the lessons you've learned and continue moving.

Reach out to your accountability partner and fill them in on what happened, so they can offer you the support you need. With time, as the distance between you and sugar grows, the cravings will diminish. However, you need to understand that if you succumb to the cries and screams of your sugar brain and go back to sugar full-time, the cravings will come back with full force too.

## KEY POINTS

Cravings are a natural and expected part of a sugar detox. Eventually, they creep up for everyone. To be successful, you will need to ensure you don't fall into the temptation that will arise from cravings.

To deal with cravings, there are many things you can do, including:

- Eat a healthy meal
- Enjoy a hot shower or bath
- Take a walk
- Drink some tea
- Practice mindfulness
- Add a bit of apple cider vinegar to your water bottle
- Get enough sleep
- Don't beat yourself up if you make a mistake. It is a part of the learning experience. Understand the lesson and get right back on track.

# PUTTING IT ALL TOGETHER

You've covered a lot of ground getting to this point, so let's go through a quick recap of everything one last time.

## CHAPTER 1: WHY SUGAR IS DESTROYING YOUR HEALTH

In this chapter, you discovered the major types of sugars: natural sugars from fruits and dairy; and refined sugar, which is the highly processed type. Broken down into its main parts, refined sugar is made up of fructose and glucose, and we consume an insane amount of it every year thanks to the modern Western diet.

Fructose is cheaper and sweeter than glucose, which

is why you can find it in almost all processed foods, usually in the form of high fructose corn syrup. Fructose, even though it's found naturally in fruit, is processed very similarly to how ethanol from alcohol is processed, by the liver. The liver, for the most part, turns fructose straight into visceral fat, the type that hugs the organs around our midsection. This can lead to a similar appearance of an alcoholic's beer belly except, in this case, it's a sugar belly.

Glucose, on the other hand, is used to fuel every cell in the body, but it cannot do that without insulin. Insulin is used by the body to open cells, so they can receive glucose as fuel. Excess glucose is converted to glycogen, which is the storage form of glucose kept in the liver and muscles. Your body reserves about a day's worth of calories as glycogen. Excess glucose beyond that is converted into fat.

Here's where things get interesting. If you have glycogen reserves available, your body will not use your fat as fuel. This is why dieting is so freakin' hard. You could be busting your butt in the gym, eating what you're "supposed" to eat, and still not lose weight. If your diet is high in carbs, even healthy carbs like fruit or whole grains, your body will keep restoring its glycogen levels and never tap into its fat storage.

And that's just one bad result of a diet of carbs and sugar:

- Sugar is what turns healthy "Pattern A" LDL cholesterol into oxidized "Pattern B" LDL cholesterol, which is what clogs arteries and leads to heart disease.
- Excess sugar intake leads to the cells of your body becoming insulin resistant, meaning your body now needs more insulin to do the same job it did before. It is this which helps lead to type 2 diabetes, and possibly dementia and Alzheimer's, which a growing number of researchers now classify as "type 3 diabetes".

## CHAPTER 2: A DRUG FOR THE WHOLE FAMILY

In this chapter, you discovered why sugar is so addictive and so hard to give up.

- **We are born to love it:** Because our ancestors got quick energy from sugar, it is embedded deep within us to love it. As soon as you taste it, the brain registers it as a pleasurable substance that we can't seem to get enough of.

- **It is very addictive**: Sugar urges your brain to release dopamine, which is a feel-good chemical, similar to what many feel during drug use. And when you no longer consume it, you can experience withdrawal symptoms similar to drug withdrawal, because your brain has become dependent on it. Not to mention, you can grow a tolerance to sugar, which means you need more and more to get the same dopamine release as you did before.

- **You can find it almost everywhere**: Processed sugar is in almost everything we consume these days—from the most obvious culprits like soda and candy, down to surprising ones like whole grain bread, rice, oatmeal, and salad dressings.

- **It causes a ravenous appetite**: Insulin, the hormone to deal with all that sugar intake, actively turns off your leptin signals so that you keep eating and never feel satisfied.

- **It causes a nasty sugar crash**: The high highs inevitably lead to low lows in your blood-sugar levels. These drastic swings cause you to feel low in energy, stressed and anxious, causing you to turn back to sugar to feel "better" again.

## CHAPTER 3: THE SWEET LIFE WITHOUT SUGAR

Giving up sugar offers you a range of benefits:

- **It is better for your skin:** Removing sugar from your diet helps you get rid of wrinkles and eye bags underneath your eyes. Because sugar creates toxic AGEs in the body, which hasten the aging process, you get to enjoy a youthful look for longer when you give up a diet high in sugar.
- **It helps you sleep better:** A no-sugar diet can help you get better sleep by ensuring you fall asleep much quicker and sleep more soundly. What's more, you wake up feeling completely refreshed instead of feeling like you have not had enough sleep.
- **Stable energy levels:** Taking sugar out of your diet can help you maintain stable

energy levels, as opposed to them constantly spiking and crashing.

- **It leads to all-around happiness:** Giving up sugar may feel like you're giving up on a source of pleasure in your life, but it's easy to forget all the other sources of pleasure that it has caused you to give up gradually over time—things like a healthy weight, heart, and liver, not to mention restful sleep, stable energy, and full control over appetite along with what you eat.

## CHAPTER 4: WHY A DETOX IS YOUR BEST OPTION

A zero sugar detox involves you doing away with all forms of sugar in your diet. This includes alternate sources of sugar such as carbs.

The plan can last anywhere from three days to 1-2 weeks, a month, or more. Your best option is dependent on what you can handle, so you need to consider your personal situation and diet carefully. I would recommend that you go for the two-week detox, as this will give you the most benefits without jumping into something intimidating like a month-long strategy. When you are done, the outcome can help determine if you want to continue with the zero sugar lifestyle.

## CHAPTER 5: WHAT TO EXPECT DURING YOUR DETOX

You will deal with withdrawal symptoms, and this is something that you can't avoid. The reality is that it gets uncomfortable before you start to enjoy all of the benefits. You've heard the saying "It gets worse before it gets better!"

You are going to experience both physical and mental withdrawal symptoms when you go into the sugar detox plan, so you have to be prepared for it.

Some of the mental symptoms you will experience include anxiety, depression, changes in sleep patterns, and concentration problems, while the physical symptoms may include headaches, fatigue, and dizziness. However, your goal is to get past these symptoms, and things will become much easier soon after.

When the sugar withdrawal symptoms come, there are ways to deal with it, including:

- Have sugar-free snacks on you at all times

- Drink lots of water, as it's easy to confuse thirst for hunger
- Work out often, so you get those feel-good endorphins going
- Get more sleep

You have to be prepared for the difficulties that go with a sugar detox. You are going to be making a change to your lifestyle, which means some of your routines may also change. Your social life may take a hit, and it might become challenging to hang out with friends or go on dates due to your limited diet. That said, it's only for the length of the detox, and the rewards that come with getting sugar out of your life are worth every inconvenience.

## CHAPTER 6: FOODS THAT WILL RUIN YOUR DETOX THE MOMENT YOU EAT THEM

There are many things you will be unable to eat during a sugar detox diet. One of the most important are foods that have a high Glycemic/Insulin Index load.

The Glycemic Index is a number that teaches you how fast your body transforms the carbohydrates in any food you consume to glucose. The following are a few ways to determine if a food item is good or bad using their GI score:

- Meals with 55 or less = Low (good)
- Meals with 56 - 69 = Medium (reasonable)
- Meals with 70 or higher = High (bad)

Also, you will need to stay away from numerous foods like:

- Sodas
- Grains
- Some fruits
- Processed/packaged meals
- Starchy veggies
- Dried fruits
- Sweetened dairy products
- Artificial sweeteners
- Condiments
- Everything that contains added sugar

You may need to go through the labels to determine the ingredients in any product you are about to consume, to ensure there is no sugar. Better still, just stop eating anything that comes in a package or box. That alone will take the majority of the guesswork out of what you can't have for the duration of your detox.

CHAPTER 7: WHAT TO EAT TO CRUSH YOUR DETOX FROM DAY 1

Your meal options will have to change for the sugar detox plan to be successful. Some of the best choices available to you include:

- **Protein:** like poultry, beans, pork, meat, and even seafood. They do not consist of sugar and are essential for your body to function at peak capacity. However, if you are going to be consuming any animal, you want to make sure they were raised with natural food and not artificial supplements.
- **Fats:** Healthy fats are an essential part of any diet, including your no-sugar diet. It does not have any impact on your blood sugar levels and is vital for your body's peak performance.
- **Vegetables:** Your vegetable options are almost limitless (minus the starchy variety), and many have little to no effect on your blood-sugar level. They offer you tons of

minerals, vitamins, fiber, and antioxidants,
all of which are great for your overall health.

Other things to consume as much as you want include legumes, nuts, and green tea, plus of course plenty of water. Lastly, herbs and spices are a great addition to help your meals feel less bland and add flavor, or in tea form for a delicious pick-me-up.

To ensure you are eating the right way during your mealtimes, make certain you do the following:

- Keep your meals simple
- Pick a protein
- Pick a fat
- Pick a vegetable or two
- Add some herbs and spices

Lastly, you want your sugar detox plan to go as seamlessly as possible. For this reason, you will want to do the following:

- Purge your kitchen
- Make a meal list
- Restock your fridge with new, healthier snacks

## CHAPTER 8: THE MOST CRUCIAL STEP: ACCOUNTABILITY

Being accountable is crucial to your sugar detox plan. Accountability means taking responsibility for your actions and ensuring you do everything to complete the goal you have set for yourself, which is staying away from sugar.

To stay accountable, there are numerous routes to take, the most important being to find an accountability partner. Ideally, it's best to choose someone neutral but who still cares about your well-being. To choose the right accountability partner, they need to have most, if not all, of the following attributes:

- Someone who does not judge
- Someone who cares about you
- Someone who knows that making mistakes is part of the process
- Someone who is not scared of calling you out when you stray

An accountability partner could be a friend, colleague or family member. It could also be someone who has gone through what you are going through presently.

Once you finally settle on an accountability partner, you should go through a few initial steps:

- Set up guidelines
- State your expectations
- Go through your goals

If you would like to add some more pressure to ensure you stick to your detox, you can make your goals public so that everyone around you can keep you in check. You can use social media to join groups and find people who have the same interests as you or choose more than one accountability partner.

## CHAPTER 9: WHEN CRAVING REARS ITS UGLY FACE

Cravings are a natural and an expected part of a sugar detox. Eventually, they creep up on for everyone. To be successful, you will need to ensure you don't fall into the temptation that will arise from cravings.

To deal with cravings, there are many things you can do, including:

- Eat a healthy meal
- Enjoy a hot shower or bath
- Take a walk
- Drink some tea
- Practice mindfulness
- Add a bit of apple cider vinegar to your water bottle
- Get enough sleep

Lastly, don't beat yourself up if you make a mistake. It is a part of the learning experience. Understand the lesson and get right back on track.

## BONUS CHAPTER: THE WIGGLE FACTOR

Well hey there! Welcome to the bonus chapter.

You either:

1. Read all the way through the book and finally made it here;
2. Started to get discouraged reading how hard this whole detox thing would be and skipped to this chapter;
3. Went straight here from the introduction as I would have.

Either way, I'm glad you're here. Letting go of sugar is no easy task, especially when you're surrounded by it and your brain literally rewards you for eating it.

I wish my brain rewarded me for eating vegetables!

Oh! And if you try to go without it, you have to feel like garbage first before you feel better.

Awesome.

Could this be any harder?!

This is where the Wiggle Factor comes in. The Wiggle Factor allows you to be less strict with your diet/detox, to still enjoy your favorite foods, and still see results. It creates the wiggle room you need to stray from your diet, to safely cave in to the temptation to eat food you're not "supposed" to eat, and not set you back.

It can even help you with your detox to get sugar completely out of your system.

It can be added to any diet, any budget, and any lifestyle.

Not only that, but it's not an exercise routine, a procedure, a pill, or anything like that.

In fact, it's nothing new. It's been around for thousands of years.

Sounds too good to be true, doesn't it?

But it's 100 percent true, and you can start adding the Wiggle Factor to your diet today.

It's so simple and yet so powerful.

Interested to find out what it is?

I bet you are.

Here's the craziest part, you're already doing it.

Just not enough to give you the wiggle room you need to make it work for you.

I've got all the details in my new book, *The Wiggle Factor*, and I want to give you a free copy as a gift for picking up your copy of *Zero Sugar Detox*.

You can go to this URL: https://fearpunchingcody.com/zerosugardetoxkit. Just tell me where to send you your free copy!

You can also simply scan this QR Code:

Or better yet, simply text DETOXSUGAR to (678) 506-7543 to download a free copy of my latest book.

And in case you're wondering, there's no catch. In all honesty, I'm simply hoping you'll enjoy it so much that you'll tell your friends about it.

And do reach out to me if *The Wiggle Factor* has helped you in any way. I'd love to hear from you!

Good luck on your sugar detox!

You can do this!

**fist bump**

—Cody

P.S. You're also going to get your Zero Sugar Detox Starter Kit!

## AFTERWORD

Congratulations! You made it to the end of the book. This is proof that you are serious about enjoying the benefits that come with getting rid of sugar from your life.

However, you need to understand that going on a no-sugar diet is not easy. You are literally altering things that you have grown accustomed to, so it's certainly going to require some hard work. Still, it doesn't mean that it can't be achieved.

So long as you follow all of the steps and strategies covered in this book, you will free yourself from sugar addiction and discover the sweeter side of life.

I don't promise that you won't face difficulties along the line. Sugar withdrawal symptoms are no joke;

the severity of your symptoms will be based on how much sugar you've been consuming. Coupled with this, there will also be cravings that you'll need to overcome.

But if you can get past all of these, you will enjoy the tons of mental and physical benefits that a sugar detox has to offer. Remember, mistakes are part of the entire process. If you make a mistake along the line, don't waste too much time blaming yourself. Instead, get back up and keep aiming for the sugar-free life you desire.

See you at the end of this journey, living the sugar-free life that you deserve.

# JOIN THE FACEBOOK GROUP!

Hey reader! You discovered in chapter 8 the importance of have the accountability to make it through this, and just how much easier things become when you have an entire community of people just like you cheering you on.

I'd like to personally invite you to our Facebook group. We're a bunch of sugar-free weirdos that have created a supported community like none other.

We share recipes, wins, mistakes, jokes (really bad jokes), and host challenges to crank up some competitive motivation.

If this sounds like something you'd be interested in,

you go to this URL to join the group: https://www.-facebook.com/groups/the.f.factor.fb.group/

Or you can even scan this QR code:

See you there!

**fist bump**

-Cody

# WHO IS CODY SMITH?

Cody Smith is a fist bumping, high-fat diet eating, intermittent fasting, ding-a-ling father of two princesses who will never date so long as he may live. He is also a bestselling author and award-winning speaker.

Cody spends embarrassingly long hours diving into nutrition and fitness research, articles, and news (along with experimenting on himself) to discovery optimum health, fitness, and weight loss tactics.

If you'd like to reach out to him (and he'd sure love it if you did), you can reach him at cody@fearpunch-ingcody.com.

**Fair warning, if he asks to hop on the phone to chat, run. He'll talk your ear off.**

# REFERENCES

About the Glycemic Index. (n.d.). Retrieved from https://www.gisymbol.com/about-glycemic-index/

Adams, R. (2017, December 7). Sugar Is Giving You Acne. No, Really. Retrieved from https://www.huffpost.com/entry/sugar-bad-for-skin_n_4071548

Couric, K. (2019, October 30). How to Quit Sugar Without Being Miserable. Retrieved from https://medium.com/wake-up-call/how-to-quit-sugar-healthy-diet-tips-fc5aee5e8cd0

Cutting out sugar: The beginner's guide. (2020, January 24). Retrieved from https://www.wellandgood.com/good-food/beginners-guide-to-cutting-out-sugar/

Forrest, C., Wong, L., DeGuzman, D., DeGuzman, D., Rowan, M., Michael, … Sam. (2019, December 27). Sugar Detox: 10 Tips to Go Sugar-Free. Retrieved from https://www.cleaneatingkitchen. com/sugar-detox-tips-sugar-free/

How Eating Sweets Affects Your Slumber and Energy. (n.d.). Retrieved from https://www.sleep. org/articles/sugar-impacts-sleep/

Hussle. (n.d.). THE BEST (ALCOHOLIC) DRINKS IF YOU ARE CUTTING OUT SUGAR. Retrieved from https://www.hussle.com/community/food/ the-best--alcoholic--drinks-to-reach-for-if-you- are-cutting-out-sugar

I can't stick to a diet for more than a few weeks. Here's why and what to do about it. (2019, September 6). Retrieved from https://www. mybodytutor.com/blog/how-to/2016/01/cant- stick-to-a-diet-heres-why-and-what-to-do-about-it

Johnson, J. (2019, December 13). No-sugar diet: 8 tips and health benefits. Retrieved from https:// www.medicalnewstoday.com/articles/319991. php#8-tips-for-cutting-out-sugar

Mason, P. (2020, February). Low Carb Down Under. Low Carb Down Under. Retrieved from https://

www.youtube.com/watch?v=
DXKJaQeteE0&t=1171s

Metrus, L. (2018, May 10). 9 Celebrity Nutritionist–
Approved Ways to Beat Your Sugar Cravings.
Retrieved from https://www.byrdie.com/how-to-
cut-sugar-cravings

Razzetti, G., & Razzetti, G. (2019, September 16).
Why An Accountability Partner Will Increases Your
Chances of Success - Gustavo Razzetti. Retrieved
from https://liberationist.org/how-to-increase-
your-chances-of-success-get-an-accountability-
partner/

This Is Your Brain on Sugar (Trust Us, It's Not Pret-
ty). (2019, August 21). Retrieved from https://www.
bulletproof.com/diet/healthy-eating/too-much-
sugar-bad-for-brain/

Van Harmelen, V., Reynisdottir, S., Eriksson, P.,
Thörne, A., Hoffstedt, J., Lönnqvist, F., & Arner, P.
(1998, June). Leptin secretion from subcutaneous
and visceral adipose tissue in women. Retrieved
from https://www.ncbi.nlm.nih.gov/
pubmed/9604868

Wbur. (2015, January 7). Is Sugar More Addictive
Than Cocaine? Retrieved from https://www.wbur.

org/hereandnow/2015/01/07/sugar-health-research

Woerner, A. (2016, July 14). The 30-Second Trick That Might Stop Your Food Cravings. Retrieved from http://dailyburn.com/life/health/30-second-trick-food-cravings-110614/

Printed in Great Britain
by Amazon

54581640R00095